# The Holistic Nutritionist's Guide to Lawful Practice in Canada

## Revised Edition

## Glenn M. Rumbell, B.A., LL.B.

**Canadian Cataloguing in Publication Data**

Rumbell, Glenn M.
The Holistic Nutritionist's Guide to Lawful Practice in Canada
Revised Edition


ISBN – 13:978-1517420567

# Preface

This book was commissioned by the Canadian Association of Natural Nutritional Practitioners (CANNP) in response to a need for a single resource for Holistic Nutritionists across Canada that summarizes the laws surrounding their profession.

The term "nutritionist" is one of those fuzzy, undefined terms that we use every day and often do not think about. In one sense, its meaning is obvious—a nutritionist is a person who knows and provides advice about nutritional well-being. But on the other hand, this definition does not tell us much, because in most areas of Canada anyone can call themselves a nutritionist, regardless of their training, experience, beliefs or manner of practice. And in provinces where its meaning is defined, and where the practice of a nutritionist is regulated, the "nutritionists" who practice there are not the ones for whom this book is written.

This book was written for unregulated, unlicensed independent nutritionists. By this I mean individuals who provide advice about nutrition to clients, but who are not members of a provincially regulated health profession because they have an alternative approach to promoting health and well-being. Individuals who view the body holistically. Individuals who believe health is not defined by the absence of disease but rather by the presence of vitality and energy. Individuals who believe natural is necessarily better. Nutritionists who believe you truly are what you eat.

The purpose of this book is to provide unlicensed nutritionists with an understanding of the major regulations that restrict what they can and cannot do in their daily practices and how they represent themselves to the public.

If you are an unlicensed nutritionist, it is crucially important that you take the time to know this.

We live in an age of increasing government regulation within the health industry and there is no single philosophical perspective that unites the regulators. The approaches governments take, from province to province and over time within a single province, vary from laisse fair to paternalistic, from supporting the right of consumers to choose, to granting select professions monopolies over whole areas of practice.

As a result, regulation in Canada is a varied landscape ranging from the open door environment of Alberta—where anyone is free to diagnose and treat diseases and disorders (provided that they do not prescribe or administer a treatment that is restricted)—to the closed door world of New Brunswick, where it is illegal for anyone but a licensed dietitian (or member of another Regulated Health Profession that is similarly empowered) to provide the service of "assessing nutritional needs of individuals and developing and implementing nutritional care plans based on the assessments."

No matter where you live and practice, it is important to know the rules that regulate what you can and cannot do. If you do, you can safely, effectively and profitably operate an unlicensed nutritionist practice in much of Canada.

I would like to thank the many people who assisted in the research and writing of this book, including my fellow directors at the Canadian Association of Natural Nutritional Practitioners, Paul Fink, Wendy Gibson and Beth Gorbet, my good friend and business partner, Martin Ross, my research assistants Meghan Parker and Justin D'Aloisio, Charlotte Rumbell for her assistance in proofing the text and the many others who reviewed and provided comments on this book. Thank you all.


Glenn Rumbell
Toronto,
July 2015

# How to Use this Book

This book has been structured to enable readers to quickly and efficiently gain an understanding of the laws in effect in their province.

Chapters 1 and 2 provide a general overview of the regulation of health service practitioners throughout Canada to provide a framework in which the laws of each province can be understood.

Chapter 3 contains summaries of the laws of each province, organized alphabetically on a province by province basis. I have also included extracts from the statutes and regulations that most directly impact unlicensed nutritionists to allow readers the opportunity to review the actual words that detail what can and cannot be done. After reading chapters 1 and 2, you should carefully review the legislative summary for your province, including these extracts.

Chapter 4 contains a discussion of the meanings of key terms that are used throughout the provincial statutes and regulations, terms such as "diagnose" and "drug" and "practice of medicine" and "treatment." It is crucial to read this chapter, as it is virtually impossible to know what a prohibition against rendering a diagnosis means, for example, unless you also know what actions have been found to constitute this activity.

The last chapter of this book is designed to enable the reader to pull everything together. In this section there are concrete recommendations on how to organize and run an unlicensed nutritional consulting practice in a way that minimizes the chances of breaching the laws of your province.

As you read this book, you will also notice that I have relied upon several stock phrases.

I have chosen to refer to unlicensed nutritionists as "**Holistic Nutritionists**" to clearly differentiate them from the licensed nutritionists who exist in some provinces as part of a combined profession of dietitians and nutritionists. The phrase "**Regulated Health Professions**" refers collectively to all health professions, (e.g., dietetics, medicine, naturopathy, etc.) that are formally regulated within a province and that require a licence to practice. To simplify matters somewhat, I refer to the various rules and regulations and policies that restrict what can and cannot be done within a province simply as "**rules**" regardless of whether they are drawn from a statute, a regulation or some other source. I have opted to use the phrase "**diseases and disorders**" to refer collectively to all diseases, disorders, conditions and abnormal states that can affect the human body, regardless of the precise language used in the rules of a particular province. However, this is a form of shorthand and in all cases the statutes and regulations of your province should be consulted for the exact language used.

When I refer to "**Restricted Activities**" I am referring to specific activities and procedures which, in certain provinces, may only be performed by members of Regulated Health Professions who are authorized to do so under that province's rules. When I refer to a province as using a "**Restricted Activity framework**" therefore, I am a stating that the province uses Restricted Activities as the primary means of regulating who may and may not provide health services. By contrast, when I state that a province uses a "**Professional Exclusivity framework**" I am stating that a province primarily regulates the provision of health services by empowering self-regulated professions, such as physicians, naturopaths and dietitians, to perform the services of their profession, usually coupled with a prohibition restricting persons outside these professions from providing such services.

# Contents

# Chapter 1
# Why Regulate?

It is often said within the Holistic Nutritionist community that the profession of a Holistic Nutritionist (and by this I mean an individual who provides nutritional consulting services to the public, but who is not a member of a Regulated Health Profession such as medicine, or dietetics, or naturopathy) is not regulated in Canada. But this is an incorrect statement.

In the area of health services, rules have long existed to ensure those who purport to diagnose and treat illnesses have the requisite skill and knowledge to do so. The reasoning for this is very straightforward and understandable—the need to protect people, when they are at their weakest and most vulnerable (and very often most desperate) from the unscrupulous and incompetent who would prey upon them. This includes both those who sell remedies to the public and those who treat the sick.

Holistic Nutritionists, like everyone else in our society, are subject to these rules.

To understand the various rules that touch upon nutrition advice it is very important to keep in mind this consumer protection mandate. I say this because it is only by understanding the reason why the rules exist that we can fully understand how they are likely to be applied. It also empowers us to recognize when a rule may exist for other, less legitimate reasons.

Webster's College Dictionary defines a *quack* to be "a fraudulent pretender of medical skill, a charlatan" and *Snake Oil* to be a "liquid concoction of questionable medical value sold as an all-purpose curative especially by travelling hucksters." The rules Holistic Nutritionists face today were largely put in place to respond to a lengthy history of quacks and sellers of snake oil.

The period from the eighteenth century to the early twentieth century was a golden era for remedies commonly known as patent medicines. These elixirs were created at a time when very little was known about the biology of health and disease causation. As a result, patent medicines typically contained no (or virtually no) effective ingredients or nutritional content. In many cases the only active agents and the ingredients that tended to make a patient feel better were drugs such as morphine and alcohol. Patent medicines also tended to be promoted aggressively through wild miracle-like curative claims.

In 1889 and 1890, for example, while an influenza epidemic raged around the world, the Carbolic Smoke Ball Company sold its product, the Carbolic Smoke Ball, as a preventive and cure for the flu as well as several other diseases. The company even offered a £100 reward to anyone who contracted the flu while using its product. Unfortunately, the device did not contain any medicinal ingredients or nutritional supplements. Instead, it consisted of a rubber ball filled with carbolic acid, which was inhaled via a tube inserted into the nose. While the fumes would cause the user's nose to run, they did absolutely nothing to prevent or cure the flu or to reinforce the immune system. When a claim on the reward was finally made by Louisa Carlill, the company at first ignored her, and then tried to dodge its obligation to pay the reward by claiming she did not use their product correctly.[1]

Another outlandish case from the turn of the century involves a tonic known as "The Microbe Killer" and marketed under the telling image of a young man using a baseball bat to bash a scythe from the boney hands of the skeleton of death. This tonic was promoted as a curative for all diseases and claimed to work by killing the microbes that cause them. At its height, The Microbe Killer was manufactured in factories across the United States, England and Australia, and sold around the world. The tonic's creator, a gardener named William Radam, became very wealthy. Once again, however, the tonic did not cure all diseases—*any diseases*—or even provide a useful injection of vitamins. Upon analysis, its composition was shown to be more than 99% water with traces of sulphuric acid and red wine.

Equally important for consumer protection is the need to ensure practitioners have the education and skill required of their profession. An unskilled person with good intentions can do as much harm as a quack who is perfectly aware of the fraud he or she is perpetrating.

The case of R. v. Kish[2] involves the activities of Robert and Margo Kish, two *phytologists* (a system of healing that combines spiritualism and nutrition) charged with unlawfully practising

---

[1] For those who are interested in such things, Mrs. Carlill won her case. The decision, which is known as Carlill v. Carbolic Smoke Ball Company [1892] EWCA Civ 1, is a landmark decision in the advancement of contract law as it relates to unilateral contracts and still studied in law schools today.

[2] R. v. Kish (1993), 12 Alta. L.R. (3d) 185

medicine. The charges against the Kishes arose from their attempt to cure their patient, Edward Pollack, of his terminal lung cancer using hydrogen peroxide (applied both internally and externally) and nutritional supplements. Such was their confidence they even purportedly counselled Mr. Pollack against taking chemotherapy and radiation treatments. Now, whatever your beliefs are about nutritional therapy, or about the use of hydrogen peroxide to fight cancer (and the court was convinced of the sincerity of the Kishes' beliefs) I think we can all agree that nutritional counsellors are overstepping their training when they emphatically claim to have a cure for terminal stage lung cancer and counsel a client to suspend all conventional medical treatments. When Mr. Pollack died within the time frame estimated by his doctor his family turned to the Kishes. They were charged and found guilty of practising medicine without a licence because they intentionally administered a treatment (hydrogen peroxide) for a disease (lung cancer).

These few examples illustrate the problem the rules are intended to address. The public needs protection from quacks and the sellers of snake oil. The difficult question is where the line is to be drawn. Draw it too loosely, people can be harmed and defrauded. Draw it too tightly, innovation and freedom of choice are stifled.

To further complicate matters, even a cursory review of the rules will tell you there is often more going on than simple consumer protection. For example, it is obvious to anyone who practices a complimentary therapy that the rules are strongly biased towards a western scientific approach to health and wellness. Practices that incorporate spiritual, eastern and other less traditional approaches are often tossed into the quack and snake oil bin. Such mainstreams practices (to many) as naturopathy and acupuncture, for example, remain outside the list of Regulated Health Professions in 4 and 5 provinces respectively. This bias has also resulted in Natural Health Products increasingly being regulated in the same manner as pharmaceuticals.

In some instances the rules also reflect the enormous power of the existing, entrenched professions. While it is unarguably legitimate consumer protection to restrict the performance of "a procedure on tissue below the dermis" (i.e., surgery) to qualified physicians as is done in Ontario, it is much harder to argue the same in respect of restricting "any treatment of any disease or ailment . . . by any form of treatment, influence or appliance . . . for hire, gain or hope of reward" as is done in Saskatchewan. In many provinces the rules appear to have, at least in part, a bias towards protecting physicians and other select professions from competition, leaving the fate of complementary therapy practitioners in such provinces to the mercy and enforcement attitude of regulators. While the arguments in support of such restrictive rules are always couched in the language of consumer protection, the impact of these rules is to create an environment of uncertainty and to lessen competition, particularly from practices outside the rubric of western science and medicine.

While googling around on this subject[3], I came across several lists of some famous (and in some circles still infamous) scientists once labelled as quacks by their peers. Included among these were Thomas Allinson, the founder of naturopathy (a Regulated Health Profession in British Columbia, Manitoba, Ontario, Saskatchewan, Alberta and Nova Scotia); Samuel Hahnemann, the founder of homeopathy (homeopathic remedies are sold throughout Canada and regulated under the Natural Health Products Regulations under Canada's *Food and Drugs Act*); D.D. Palmer, the founder of chiropractory (a Regulated Health Profession in all Canadian provinces); Louis Pasteur, who among other things, confirmed the germ theory of disease; Linus Pauling, a Nobel Prize winner in chemistry who was widely ridiculed for advocating the use of large doses of vitamin C to fight the common cold and the father of orthomolecular medicine; and most recently Mehmet Oz a renowned heart surgeon and popular TV personality (The Dr. Oz Show) who has been accused of promoting pseudoscientific health treatments and supplements, and even called before the United States Senate.

Many of these innovators found their ability to make advances in healthcare available to the public frustrated by accusations of quackery and professional shunning.

Today, Holistic Nutritionists and practitioners of other complimentary therapies face similar challenges. In most provinces a Holistic Nutritionist is prohibited from making a diagnosis and treating diseases and disorders. This can even include something as obvious as diagnosing obesity and recommending treatment through a change in diet. Where this is the case it is fair to argue that the rules are too restrictive, that innovation and progress are being frustrated, and that government regulation may perhaps exist more to protect existing professional monopolies, big pharma and the western scientific method, than to protect the public.

For Holistic Nutritionists the key to fighting over regulation is to educate the public and regulators about the role of complementary therapies, and the right of consumers to make informed choices, while respecting the need for clear rules to protect consumers from fraud and other harmful practices. In the mean time they must be very careful about what they do.

---

[3] Special thanks to the contributors to "Quackery," *Wikipedia: The Free Encyclopedia* [online]. Wikimedia Foundation, Inc. [Accessed June 2, 2015.] <http://en.wikipedia.org/wiki/Quackery>.

# Chapter 2
# Overview of Regulation in Canada

Canada is a federation of provinces and territories. This means the rules that govern our lives are promulgated by the federal and various provincial governments within each of their areas of jurisdiction and by our cities and municipalities within the jurisdictions that have been delegated to them. As a result, the regulation of health services in Canada is in many ways a patchwork quilt, with significant differences existing among our various provinces and regions.

The provision of health services to the public is primarily regulated by provincial governments. This means the task of describing what a Holistic Nutritionist can and cannot do in Canada must be done on a province-by-province basis. What may be lawful in Alberta, for example, may result in a fine or even imprisonment if practiced in Nova Scotia. In the next chapter the reader will find legislative summaries for each of the provinces setting out the rules that impact on the ability of Holistic Nutritionists to provide nutritional advice to clients.

Within Canada, there are essentially two approaches used to regulate the provision of health services: (1) professional exclusivity—where the rules prohibit anyone other than members of a profession from carrying on the business and practice of that profession (e.g., only members of the provincial College of Physicians may practice medicine); and (2) restricted activities— where the rules create a list of defined activities and procedures that may only be performed by members of Regulated Health Professions granted the authority to do so (e.g., only members of the provincial College of Physicians may reset or cast a bone fracture).

## Regulating by Professional Exclusivity

The first approach, which I call the Professional Exclusivity framework, is the traditional approach used for regulating health services. Historically, this approach began with the recognition of the medical profession as a discrete profession and the delegation to it of the right and obligation to regulate its own standards and members, the theory essentially being that medicine is a highly specialized activity and members of the profession are in a better position than the public to know the qualifications and standards that should apply to practitioners.[4]

Over the years the concept of what constituted the practice of medicine fragmented as new health practices emerged and specialties within the traditional field of medicine developed and splintered off. Eventually, many of these new health professions sought the prestige and benefits of professional status and petitioned governments for the right of self-governance. Today, somewhere between twenty and thirty health professions are recognized and granted the right of self-regulation within most provinces.

While this approach to regulation appears simple, it actually can lead to confusion because these statutes often do not properly define the activities that constitute the practice of the profession they regulate, instead leaving this task to the governing body of the profession itself and the courts.

Using the practice of medicine as an example, common sense should tell us that performing surgery, setting broken bones, diagnosing a disease such as cancer and prescribing and administering chemotherapy as a treatment involves the practice of medicine. But what about less obvious activities? What about determining whether a person is obese and structuring a treatment? Diagnosing obesity is relatively easy. It can be done with little more evidence than our eyes, and the treatment for it (exercise and diet) is also pretty straightforward. Yet, obesity is also a recognized disease. Does the act of identifying and treating obesity constitute the practice of medicine? To take this argument to its extreme, what about dehydration and starvation? If I tell a dehydrated person to drink water or a starving person to eat food, am I diagnosing and treating a condition? What if I recommend they take vitamins?

For Holistic Nutritionists who want to ensure they do not cross the line and face a charge of unlawfully practising medicine this grey zone is a real problem.

In Canada, the provinces of New Brunswick, Newfoundland and Labrador, Nova Scotia, Prince Edward Island and Saskatchewan currently regulate the provision of health services

---

[4] Casey, J. T., *The Regulation of Professions in Canada* (Toronto: Carswell, 1988).

using this approach[5]. Holistic Nutritionists operating within these provinces must comply with all of the various statutes and regulations that create the twenty or thirty odd Regulated Health Professions within their province of residence.

Most schools that educate and train Holistic Nutritionists teach that the practice of Holistic Nutrition involves the assessment and promotion of health and wellness. When faced with clients in ill health, however, it can be very tempting to move beyond this and to start diagnosing and/or treating suspected and known conditions. As a result, it is particularly important for Holistic Nutritionists to understand the boundaries of Regulated Health Professions whose professional practices include the diagnosis of diseases and disorders and the use of nutrition and supplements both as treatments and to promote health. Of particular concern, therefore, are the statutes and regulations that define the professional practice of medicine, which is both regulated and restricted in all provinces, dietetics, which is regulated in all provinces, but only restricted in some, and naturopathy, which is regulated and restricted only in some provinces.

In the next chapter I have included summaries of key provisions from these statutes, organized on a province-by-province basis, for easy reference.

## Regulating by Restricted Activities

The other regulatory approach taken by Canadian provinces, which I call the Restricted Activities framework, involves focusing more directly on consumer protection by controlling who may perform specific defined acts and procedures that are viewed to be inherently risky and therefore requiring a requisite level of skill and training to perform. For example, section 4(1) of Schedule 7.1 to the Alberta *Government Organization Act* provides in part:

> s. 4(1) No person shall perform a restricted activity or a portion of it on or for another person unless:
>
>     (a)    the person performing it
>
>         (i)    is a regulated member as defined in the Health Professions Act, and is authorized to perform it by the regulations under the *Health Professions Act . . .*

The list of Restricted Activities is defined in section 2(1) of the same schedule and provides in part:

---

[5] I have not included the province of Manitoba in this group as it is in the process of transitioning to a Restricted Activities framework.

s. 2(1)  The following, carried out in relation to or as part of providing a health service, are restricted activities:

(a)   to cut a body tissue, to administer anything by an invasive procedure on body tissue or to perform surgical or other invasive procedures on body tissue

(i)   below the dermis or the mucous membrane or in or below the surface of the cornea;

(ii)   in or below the surface of teeth, including scaling of teeth;

Regulation through a Restricted Activities framework represents the emerging trend among Canadian provinces. At the present time, the provinces of, Alberta, B.C., Ontario and Quebec have implemented Restricted Activity regulatory regimes and the province of Manitoba is in the midst of making the transition to one. This approach is now being favoured because it addresses the reality that many health professions have practice areas that both overlap and include procedures that can be safely and economically performed by unregulated professionals. In a consultation document prepared by the Government of Manitoba, the effect and benefit of moving to a "Reserved Act" (i.e., Restricted Activity) approach was described as follows:

Actions or clinical procedures that may present a demonstrable risk of harm to the public will be regulated. Many of the reserved acts can be performed by more than one profession, so collaborative care will be encouraged. These acts and procedures will be restricted to specified practitioners, so unregulated practitioners will only be able to provide them if authorized under the legislation, e.g., under delegation from a regulated health profession. Unregulated practitioners will be able to provide services that do not include reserved acts. This model will help improve patient safety.[6]

This trend is good news for Holistic Nutritionists. In provinces that have moved to a Restricted Activity framework, there is generally[7] more room to practice than in provinces where regulation occurs through professional exclusivity. In addition, because the Restricted Activities are clearly described in the rules, there is less doubt about what Holistic Nutritionists can and cannot do.

This said, the world for Holistic Nutritionists in the Restricted Activities provinces is still not perfect. Many will find the rules against diagnosing and treating diseases and disorders, which

---

[6] Health Professions Regulatory Reform Consultation Document, Proposed Umbrella Health Professions Legislation: the *Regulated Health Professions Act,* Government of Manitoba, January 2009.

[7] The province of Quebec, which aggressively enforces its prohibition against 'prescribing treatment' is a notable exception to this rule.

exist to varying degrees in the different provinces, both unnecessary and too broadly defined. Borrowing from an earlier example, are you "treating" an illness by telling a client to take vitamins to remedy a deficiency? As well, there are some fairly significant differences among the provinces about what procedures are restricted. In Alberta, for example, neither the diagnosis nor treatment of a disease or disorder is a Restricted Activity. In Ontario, the diagnosis of a disease in circumstances "in which it is reasonably foreseeable that the individual or his or her personal representative will rely on the diagnosis" is restricted, but the treatment of a previously diagnosed diseases or disorder is not. In Quebec, both the diagnosis and treatment of a disease and disorders are Restricted Activities and aggressively enforced.

In the next chapter I have included summaries of key provisions of these rules, organized on a province-by-province basis, for easy reference.

## Use of Titles

As part of regulating health professions and/or activities that are restricted and may only be performed by specified Regulated Health Professions, the provinces also restrict the use of professional titles, essentially reserving the use of titles typically associated with a profession, for the exclusive use of its members. The principle behind this is, obviously, consumer protection. If the primary purpose of regulating a profession is to ensure the quality of practitioners, it makes sense to ensure those practitioners can be readily identified by the public. An exclusive title does this.

In Canada, most provinces generally reserve titles such as "Doctor" and "Physician" and "Surgeon" and associated abbreviations for use by members of one or more of the "medical" professions (e.g., medicine, dentistry, psychiatry, etc.). In Alberta this restrictive list extends to approximately 75 specific specialties of medicine. In provinces in which naturopathy is a Regulated Health Profession, use of titles such as "Naturopath" and "Naturopathic Doctor" are similarly restricted.

The use of the title "Dietitian" is generally reserved for use by registered dietitians in all provinces. In three provinces, Alberta, Nova Scotia and Quebec, the title "Nutritionist" and/or "Registered Nutritionist" is also reserved. In addition, several provinces restrict the use of any other title or claim that may wrongly indicate a person is a member of a provincially Regulated Health Profession.

Where a title is reserved for use by one or more Regulated Health Professions, it is unlawful for a person who is not a member of one of those professions to use the title. Since there are wide differences among the provinces about which titles are reserved for use by the various

Regulated Health Professions, it is very important to check the rules that exist in your province.

In the next chapter I have included summaries of the key rules relating to the use of professional titles, organized on a province-by-province basis, for easy reference.

## Prosecution of Holistic Nutritionists

In working with Holistic Nutritionists over the years, I have noticed the existence of a popular belief that Holistic Nutritionists are frequently prosecuted (I should almost say persecuted) for doing little more than providing sound nutritional advice to their clients. If this were the case, there should be a significant body of case law (i.e., reported court decisions) that can be used to define the appropriate scope of practice and the point(s) at which a Holistic Nutritionist's actions may cross the line into the areas of medicine, naturopathy, or dietetics.

To my surprise, I could not locate a single reported case in Canada of a Holistic Nutritionist being charged with unlawful practice of medicine, naturopathy or dietetics. I located only two hybrid cases involving nutritional counselling in conjunction with other activities and one case involving a homeopath providing services that, in part, are sometimes provided by Holistic Nutritionists.

Concerned that my research was somehow missing the mark, I contacted several provincial regulatory colleges, including the Colleges of Physicians and Surgeons of Ontario, British Columbia, Quebec and Saskatchewan, to obtain their perspective on the prosecution of Holistic Nutritionists.

A representative of the College of Physicians and Surgeons of Ontario told me its jurisdiction extended only to its members, and that they forwarded any complaints (which they rarely received) about non-members to the local police. From there, I followed up with both the Ontario Provincial Police and Toronto Policc. The Toronto Police were unable (or unwilling) to refer me to a desk within their organization that would handle such a complaint. A detective with the Ontario Provincial Police confirmed his desk would deal with this issue, but he told me he could not remember a single incident of investigating and charging a Holistic Nutritionist. When asked what I should take from this, I was informed that it didn't mean it didn't happen, as he could not speak for the entire force, but that, obviously, such incidences were extremely rare. Why? The officer surmised that individuals who seek out complimentary therapy practitioners tended not to complain when those services did not comply with medical standards, and that without a complaint there is nothing to investigate.

This perspective was echoed by a representative of the Colleges of Physicians and Surgeons of Saskatchewan who informed me the College had formally adopted a policy of respecting the right of consumers to choose their own health services modality, in part, as a result of the difficulty of proceeding against complimentary therapy practitioners where clients refused to cooperate. I was told the College now focuses its efforts on cases of fraud (e.g., impersonation of a doctor) and where the service provider causes injury to the patient.

By contrast, the representative of the Quebec College of Physicians and Surgeons with whom I spoke said the Quebec College is very active in protecting consumers and prosecuting individuals for wrongful practice of medicine. But their concern was with anyone who was not a member of a Regulated Health Profession, which includes Holistic Nutritionists in Quebec but also naturopaths and others. I was referred to a Brief[8] prepared by the College of Physicians of Quebec in 1993 that is still referred to as embodying the College's view on alternative therapies:

> Most Quebec physicians, without fanfare and without masquerading under the "holistic" title have for a long time treated their patient as a whole person (global approach). Many "alternative therapies" parade under the holistic concept banner. . . . "Alternative therapies" for the most part, have not been proven scientifically or claim to be untestable by the usual scientific methods.

So what do the results of my legal research and informal enquiries mean?

First, I suspect the paucity of reported cases indicates Holistic Nutritionists are not being singled out and prosecuted (or persecuted) for unlawful practice of medicine. Second, I suspect it indicates that most Holistic Nutritionists are practising within the laws of their province and are not generally engaged in diagnosing or treating diseases or misusing professional titles. Third, I suspect it indicates enforcement is often practiced informally through the use of warnings and fines, at least in instances where no one has been harmed by the Holistic Nutritionist's actions. Finally, and most importantly, I suspect it means most Holistic Nutritionists are providing safe, useful advice to clients who are seeking a different path to wellness than that offered by traditional medicine.

So turning now to the cases I did find, what can they tell us?

The first of these cases is R. v. Kish, the facts of which I briefly summarized in Chapter 1. This case involved two phytologists, Robert and Margo Kish, who were charged with the unlawful

---

[8] Brief on Alternative Therapies, 1993. Submitted by the College of Physicians of Quebec to the Commission of Social Affairs.

practice of medicine contrary to s. 76(1)(a) of the Alberta *Medical Profession Act*[9] for prescribing hydrogen peroxide and nutritional supplements to treat the terminal lung cancer of their client, Mr. Ed Pollack.

The court's decision turned on section 77(1) of the Act, which defined the practice of medicine to include the prescription or administration of any treatment "for the prevention, alleviation or cure of any human disease, ailment, deformity, defect or injury." So the key question for the court was whether their activities constituted a "treatment" of a "human disease, ailment, deformity, defect or injury." The brother of the deceased (who had attended at the home of the Kishes with the deceased) testified that the Kishes ridiculed the medical profession, counselled against radiation and chemotherapy, and assured the deceased that they could cure his cancer.

For their part, the Kishes testified that as phytologists they devised programs for their clients that combined spiritual, mental and nutritional elements. They also argued that they had not been told of the extent of Ed Pollack's cancer. The judge summarized their testimony as follows:

> Robert Kish stated that their approach was to look at the whole body and to try and devise a program to deal with the needs of the whole person. He did go so far as to admit that "where there is a weakness within the system we try to regenerate that." With respect to the hydrogen peroxide therapy he indicated that the theory was that it was an "oxygenator" and it would also give a boost of energy and that they recommend a regime of vitamins and minerals with the hydrogen peroxide program to deal with what they thought was a small cancerous spot on his lung.

From this passage, it appears the Kishes were arguing they did not treat diseases per se but rather the whole person, with the goal of moving their clients toward wellness, which seems fairly close to the goals of a Holistic Nutritionist and an argument a Holistic Nutritionist might make about his or her own practice.

The court found the Kishes guilty of unlawfully practising medicine. Interestingly, it was not the prescription of vitamins and minerals or even an intravenous injection of B12 they gave Mr. Pollack that proved to be the problem. The court did not appear to be concerned with their efforts to boost Mr. Pollack's overall health and did not even evaluate whether such activities constituted a treatment. Instead, the smoking gun was the prescription of the hydrogen peroxide and their claim that it was a cure.

---

[9] This statute is no longer in force, having been replaced by *The Health Professions Act*.

> On the basis of all of the evidence there is no doubt in my mind that what the Kishes did was prescribe a course of treatment clearly directed at and purporting to be able to cure the cancer that Pollock suffered from. By whatever definition of "treatment" is used (and I would refer specifically to those definitions used by Cooke J. in *R. v. Ringrose* (1989), 94 A.R. 350 (Q.B.), at p. 353) the prescribing of hydrogen peroxide to be taken internally for the purpose of killing cancer cells and curing cancer falls squarely within even the narrowest interpretation of "treatment."

While it was not addressed by the court, one has to wonder whether the outcome would have been the same had the Kishes refrained from interfering with their client's chemotherapy treatments and limited their activity to providing a complimentary therapy alongside Mr. Pollack's medical treatment.

The other quasi-nutritionist case I was able to uncover was R. v. Windrum,[10] a decision of the Saskatchewan court of Queen's Bench, involving the appeal of Mr. Windrum from a charge of unlawfully practising medicine contrary to the Saskatchewan *Medical Profession Act*.

The facts of this case are in many ways (with one major exception) similar to the experiences many Holistic Nutritionists have every day. The accused did not claim or pretend to be a doctor. The client (or more accurately the mother of the client, since the actual patient was an infant girl) was also aware that the treatments recommended by Mr. Windrum were typically different than those prescribed by doctors. Mr. Windrum examined the infant physically, enquired into her medical history, drew blood from the infant girl's finger and examined it under a microscope. He diagnosed the girl as suffering from "parasites, liver impairment, liver damage, liver stress, yeast problems, deficient bone marrow, overactive spleen, inflamed spleen, genetically weak bladder, pre-cancerous condition, lymph congestion, and genetic heart condition" largely on the basis of his analysis of the blood sample.

Mr. Windrum was charged with breaching the Saskatchewan *Medical Profession Act* for diagnosing each of these conditions and for treating the infant girl by prescribing iron supplements, vitamins and other substances. Under the *Medical Profession Act* both diagnosing and treating a disease or disorder were deemed to be the practice of medicine.

For Holistic Nutritionists there are two aspects of this case that, I believe, are of particular interest.

---

[10] R. v. Windrum, [1995] 2 W.W.R. 226

First, Mr. Windrum tried to argue that as he did not hold himself out to be a doctor and did not claim to practice medicine, he could not be found to have practiced medicine. The court ruled his intentions to be irrelevant:

> Windrum argued that his acts were either not intended or not perceived as practising medicine. In my view that is not relevant. The issue before the court is whether he was practising medicine. In other words, was he diagnosing or treating patients.

Second, in deciding whether Mr. Windrum diagnosed and/or treated a disease, the court turned to a physician as an expert witness and accepted his assessment that both Mr. Windrum's diagnosis and treatment conformed to procedures that could be followed within medicine:

> Dr. Loewen, who was qualified as an expert, said that the diagnosis is a conclusion about the patient's condition based on her history, physical examination and tests if necessary. He went on to state that one can diagnose by examining the patient's blood. Furthermore, many of the conditions found by Windrum could be diagnosed by following the above process. In Dr. Loewen's opinion it was common practice to treat patients by prescribing vitamins or iron supplements.

It is not surprising that Mr. Windrum was found to have provided a diagnosis. He clearly examined his patient, including through a blood test, and provided a detailed list of conditions and ailments detected. And perhaps it is not surprising that the court found the simple prescription of vitamins and supplements to constitute administering a treatment, as they were prescribed in response to the conditions diagnosed. But it is also clear in this case that the court did not like or respect Mr. Windrum, and it is possible that this impacted on the court's willingness to find the prescription of vitamins to be administering a treatment. In commenting on the reasonableness of the sentence ($5,000 in fines) the court noted:

> In this case Windrum's actions were improper and unethical. After obtaining the trust of Loni and her mother he then attempted, without any training or expertise, to diagnose Loni. After frightening both Loni and her mother by claiming that the child suffered from many serious medical conditions, he then sought to profit from his actions.

> Windrum is a danger to the public and therefore any sentence imposed must reflect both general and individual deterrence. In my view the sentences imposed are entirely appropriate and therefore the sentence appeal is also dismissed.

The final case I uncovered and that is of interest is R. v. Sandhar,[11] an appeal decision of the Alberta court of Queen's Bench, overturning a charge against Mr. Sandhar, a homeopath, of

---

[11] R. v. Sandhar (1988), 86 A.R. 241

unlawfully practising medicine. Mr. Sandhar was charged with breaching sections 76 and 77 of the Alberta *Medical Profession Act*, which as we saw in the Kish case deemed the practice of medicine to include claiming the ability to diagnose and/or treat diseases and disorders, and administering treatment.

What is of particular interest for Holistic Nutritionists is that the diagnostic procedures and treatment prescribed by Mr. Sandhar were not the kind that would be prescribed by a typical medical physician. In fact, his diagnostic process—which centred on body energy levels—is similar to the practice of muscle testing used by many Holistic Nutritionists, and his treatments—an herbal supplement and a liver cleanser—are of the type recommended by many Holistic Nutritionists daily.

The facts are clearly set out in this extract from the decision:

> On April 23, 1985, Peggy Lewis attended the Respondent's clinic in Edmonton and told him that she had a feeling of tiredness and sluggishness, occasional backache and shortness of breath. Following Dr. LeRiche's instructions, she indicated that her doctor was thinking of examining her for thyroid problems. The Respondent had Miss Lewis fill out a questionnaire and inquired about her lifestyle and diet. He then carried out what he called an "Alert Test." The machine that was used had one rod connected to it which was placed in one of Miss Lewis' hands. This rod was moistened with a compound. Another rod was connected to a machine and the Respondent conducted an examination of Miss Lewis by touching various spots on her fingernails and toes.

> The Respondent testified that the readings from the machine indicated that Miss Lewis had possible lung congestion. The circulation reading was low which accounted for Miss Lewis having cold extremities. His testing also indicated that there was an inflammation of the liver and kidneys. It was the Respondent's belief that there was a build up of toxins which would be the cause of her tiredness and sluggishness.

> The Respondent had Miss Lewis purchase from him two bottles of drugs, one which was said to be a liver cleanser which would help her liver problems and the other was Camphora which was to alleviate the feelings of tiredness.

> Miss Lewis was charged $30.00 for a consultation fee, $10.00 for the liver cleanser and $5.00 for the Camphora.

Concerning the mysterious machine used to diagnose Ms. Lewis:

The Alert Test machine that was used by the Respondent was said by the Respondent to be used to determine a person's state of health as a precautionary measure but has nothing to do with homoeopathy. The Respondent stated the machine is designed to measure the flow of energy of various organs from acqua pressure meridian points and is a test technique he was trained in by the Society of Ultramolecular medicine in Las Vegas.

Mr. Sandhar was ultimately found to have practiced medicine in breach of the Alberta *Medical Act*. In reaching this decision, it did not matter to the court that Mr. Sandhar was following a discipline that was different from conventional western medicine, because the Act deemed even the making of a claim to diagnose illness and the act of prescribing a treatment to be within the scope of the practice of medicine.

I would like you to draw the following key points from this review of Canada's regulatory framework.

- Holistic Nutritionists are subject to extensive regulation.

- Some provinces regulate the provision of health services using a Professional Exclusivity framework in which health practices are defined (e.g.,the practice of medicine) and restricted to licensed members of that profession. This approach to regulation is the more traditional approach, but also creates the most uncertainty, as it can be difficult to know what activities make up the restricted practice.

- Some provinces regulate the provision of health services using a Restricted Activities framework in which a list of specific activities and procedures are defined to be risky, and restricted to licensed members of designated Regulated Health Professions. This approach to regulation is the more modern approach and generally enables individuals who are not members of a Regulated Health Profession to know, with a much higher degree of certainty, what activities can and cannot lawfully be performed.

- As part of regulatory framework all provinces identify and restrict the use of certain professional titles, such as "Doctor" and "Dietitian" and even "Nutritionist" for example, to one or more Regulated Health Professions.

- Anecdotal evidence indicates that Holistic Nutritionists are not being widely prosecuted for carrying on activities reserved for members of Regulated Health Professions or that constitute the practice of medicine. Among other things, this may indicate that any breaches are being enforced informally through warnings and that most Holistic

Nutritionists are providing safe complementary therapies to their clients. However, different provinces apply different standards to enforcement. A lawyer should always be consulted before commencing a practice.

- In the provinces that regulate using the Professional Exclusivity framework, Holistic Nutritionists must be careful not to diagnose diseases or disorders or to recommend treatments for diseases or disorders, as both activities comprise activities that are typically found to be part of the practice of medicine.

- If you do face a charge of unlawfully practicing medicine, (1) advising your client that you are not a physician, (2) rendering a diagnosis or recommending a treatment that is outside the scope of a common medical practice, or (3) claiming to treat the entire person, rather than the underlying condition, will not be valid defences if you are found in fact to have diagnosed an illness or prescribed a treatment.

# Chapter 3
# Provincial Rules & Regulations

The purpose of this chapter is to review the rules that restrict the right of Holistic Nutritionists to carry on a conventional practice, which for my purposes I define to mean assessing the health of paying clients and recommending dietary changes, food and nutritional supplements to improve health or address known diseases and conditions.

As mentioned in the last chapter, since this book is intended for use by individuals who are not members of a Regulated Health Profession, this goal must be achieved by way of subtraction. Meaning, since there are no rules stipulating what Holistic Nutritionists may do, we must instead look at what they are prohibited from doing. While this may seem a simple way of proceeding, it does carry with it a serious procedural difficulty. In Canada there are literally thousands of statutes regulating what we can and cannot do, and investigating, assessing and summarizing all of these would fill volumes.

Out of necessity I have, therefore, established a few ground rules to narrow the scope of my enquiry and to keep my discussion on point. In using this book the reader must keep in mind that it is not an exhaustive study of all rules that impact upon a Holistic Nutritionist's practice. Rather, it is a summary of the laws that restrict or prohibit the activities of a normal practice, along the lines of my definition at the start of this chapter.

So what are these ground rules?

First, I have (with two exceptions in respect of Alberta and Ontario) restricted my focus to reviewing rules that exist in respect to the three Regulated Health Professions that most overlap with the practice of Holistic Nutritionists: medicine, dietetics and naturopathy. The reason for looking at the practices of medicine and naturopathy is obvious. Both of these professions involve assessing health, diagnosing illness and disease and prescribing treatments that may include nutrition. Historically, medicine can also be thought of as the "root" health profession. By this I mean, the imposition of rules on what the unlicensed world can and cannot do with respect to diagnosing and treating human diseases and conditions began with medicine, and it remains the largest and most broadly defined professional practice area in health.

I have included dietetics for the obvious reason that this profession is the "Regulated Health Profession" in all provinces for nutritional advisors.[12]

As the reader may appreciate, this means I have not looked at and will not be discussing many other health professions such as nursing, massage therapy, chiropractory, etc. all of which are regulated in one or more and in most cases all provinces. And the various provincial statutes that regulate them (at least in the provinces that do not regulate using the "Restricted Activities" approach discussed in the last chapter) may restrict persons who are not licensed from practising these professions. However, it is also my assumption that such professions are sufficiently dissimilar to the practice of Holistic Nutrition that a well-intentioned and formally educated Holistic Nutritionist is not likely to accidently lapse into their practice. If, however, your practice does include advice and procedures that go beyond assessing wellness and providing nutritional advice, you should investigate the rules that apply to these and other Regulated Health Professions in your province.

Second, I have limited my scope to statutes that relate to whether a Holistic Nutritionist can carry on a conventional practice. Accordingly, I have not reviewed or summarized the many statutes of general application that might regulate how (rather than whether) these services are provided.

For example, many provinces maintain statutes that specifically regulate the collection, storage, use, release and disposal of personal information and client records. In Ontario, for example, the applicable statute is the *Personal Health Information Protection Act*, and it does apply to both regulated and unregulated health professionals. And all Canadians must comply with the federal government's *Personal Information Protection and Electronic Documents Act* (PIPEDA) which establishes rules for the collection, use and disclosure of personal

---

[12] On its web site, http://www.dieteticregulation.ca/en/whatis.php (accessed June 2, 2015), The Alliance of Canadian Dietetic Regulatory Bodies described a Registered Dietitian as follows: "A Registered Dietitian is a uniquely trained member of the health team with expertise in food and nutrition. Dietitians provide information about diet and diet therapies in the prevention and treatment of disease. Dietitians specialize in many different areas of practice including nutrition support (nutrition fed by special means such as intravenous lines and feeding tubes), education, research, and population health.

information by private organizations in the course of commercial activities. Provinces also have statutes regulating the dispensing of drugs, the preparation, storage and sale of food, and a host of other matters that may be of interest to a Holistic Practitioner depending upon the scope of his or her business.

To further complicate the regulatory landscape, it must also be remembered that regions and municipalities have the authority to regulate businesses that operate within their borders and may require someone who wants to carry on an otherwise lawful business to obtain a licence. In the city of Toronto, for example, the municipal code requires anyone who provides "Holistic Services" (which is defined to include any modality used as a tool for therapeutic and wellness purposes other than body rubs and services provided by members of Regulated Health Professions) and any location at which Holistic Services are provided, to be licensed.

These rules and many others must also be complied with, and I recommend that a lawyer who is licensed to practice in your province be consulted before opening your practice so you are aware of them.

Finally, I have not investigated or summarized laws of general application such as the Criminal Code, (which may be a factor, if you are charged with fraud) but which apply to all of us equally, regardless of whether we carry on a health services business.

By omitting all of these areas of enquiry, I am not claiming they are not relevant and have no bearing on the operation of an unregistered, unlicensed nutritional health practice. Such statutes are very relevant and must be complied with and you should always consult a lawyer to ensure you comply. However, the review of all of their implications across ten different provinces of Canada is simply a task that is beyond the scope of this book.

Now a few comments about what is included in this chapter.

In the pages that follow I have set out extracts from the key statutes and regulations that restrict the provision of health services organized on a province-by-province basis. To review the rules for a particular province, simply turn to the summary for that province. If you are not familiar with reading statutory provisions, you may find the language sometimes difficult to follow. To enable readers to focus on the most salient provisions I have tried to ease your path by omitting sub-sections and sub-clauses I deemed unnecessary for your understanding of the main rule. In many places this editing results in a discontinuity in the section numbers (.e.g., (4) followed by (7)). When you see this you can assume the numbering reflects the numbering from the statute being cited, and not a typographical error.

As previously mentioned, some provinces regulate the provision of health services by using a Restricted Activities framework. Where this is the case, these activities may not be performed except (1) by a member of a Regulated Health Profession whose members are expressly authorized to do so (typically, members of the medical profession are authorized to perform all or nearly all Restricted Activities, while members of other Regulated Health Professions are authorized to perform a subset of activities, or none at all), or (2) the situation falls within one of the limited exceptions set out in the rules. These exceptions differ from province to province but generally include providing the service under the immediate supervision of a person who is authorized to perform the activity in question, as part of spiritual counselling, or as emergency first aid. As these exceptions do not create an exception for provision of nutritional advice, I have not included them in my summaries.

In reviewing the rules, the reader will come across terms and phrases such as "practice of medicine" and "diagnose" and "treatment" that are either not or only superficially defined. In Chapter 4, I review how the courts and other legal authorities have defined some of these terms, to provide greater insight into their meaning.

I have included in the legislative summaries information concerning the use of professional titles. For expediency, I have not summarized the professional titles reserved for physicians and naturopaths, as these titles (Physician, Doctor, MD, Naturopath, etc.) are not descriptive of or typically associated with the provision of nutritional health advice, and therefore, are not likely to be used accidentally by a well-intentioned Holistic Nutritionist. So my review centres on titles reserved for use by registered dietitians.

Finally, it must always be remembered that the rules I have cited in this book are subject to change at any time and therefore cannot be relied upon to be complete, accurate or even in force at the time of reading. For certainty, the reader should always consult a lawyer or the actual statutes and regulations in place within his or her province at the time the information is required.

## Alberta

The provision of health services in Alberta is regulated using a Restricted Activity framework. The rules that impact the practices of Holistic Nutritionists are primarily found in the *Health Professions Act* and Schedule 7.1 to the *Government Organization Act*.

The *Health Professions Act* establishes the various Regulated Health Professions and the rules that apply to their operation as self-governing professions. Section 2 of Schedule 7.1 to the *Government Organization Act* establishes the Restricted Activities that may be performed only by members of designated Regulated Health Professions. A person who is not a member of a designated Regulated Health Profession may not perform any of these procedures. Interestingly, the activities of diagnosing diseases and disorders and providing treatment are not restricted, per se. So Holistic Nutritionists in Alberta are permitted to diagnose and treat diseases and disorders provided they do not perform a specific activity (e.g., prescribing drugs) that is restricted. The unlawful practice of a Restricted Activity can result in a fine of up to $5,000 for a first offence.

Under section 46 *Health Professions Act* you are required to register (i.e., be a member of a Regulated Health Profession) if you meet the education, experience and other qualifications of a Regulated Health Profession and intend to provide the services of that profession to the public. So, for example, if someone meets the requirements of The College of Dietitians of Alberta to be a Registered Dietitian and Nutritionist and wishes to provide the services of a Dietitian and Nutritionist[13] to the public, that person must become a member of the college. Failing to do so constitutes a breach of the Act and may result in a fine of $2,000 for a first offence.

Section 128 of the Health Professions Act makes it an offence to wrongly use a title that is reserved for members of a Regulated Health Profession, to falsely imply you are a member of a Regulated Health Profession, or to use "registered" or "regulated" when you are not a

---

[13] Schedule 23 "Profession of Registered Dietitians and Registered Nutritionists" to the *Health Professions Act* allows registered Dietitians and registered nutritionists to do one or more of the following:
(a)   assess nutritional status and develop, implement and evaluate food and nutrition strategies and interventions to promote health and treat illness,
(b)   apply food and nutrition principles to the management of food service systems and to the development and analysis of food and food products,
(c)   promote optimal health, food security and food safety through the development and delivery of food and nutrition education, programs and policies,
(c.1) teach, manage and conduct research in the science, techniques and practice of dietetics, and
(d)   provide restricted activities authorized by the regulations.

member of a Regulated Health Profession. Schedule 23 of the Health Professions Act reserves the titles "Nutritionist" and "Registered Nutritionist" (among others) for exclusive use by members of The College of Dietitians. The use of other variations of nutritionist, such as 'nutritional' and 'nutrition' either on their own or in combination with words other than "Registered" or "Regulated" is, strictly speaking, permitted. However, because the Health Professions Act contains rules against using a title that wrongly implies you are a member of a Regulated Health Profession you should consult with a local lawyer to ensure your use of such words does not breach this standard. The unlawful use of a professional title can result in a fine of up to $2,000 for a first offence.

A Holistic Nutritionist who is not a member of a Regulated Health Profession in Alberta may carry on a conventional nutritional practice provided he or she: (1) is not required to become a member of the College of Dietitians of Alberta by virtue of meeting the requirements of the College for registration: (2) does not perform a Restricted Activity described in Schedule 7.1 of the Government Organization Act; (3) does not market themselves to the public using a title reserved for registered dietitians, or any another Regulated Health Profession; and (4) otherwise complies with laws of general application.

## Restrictions on Activities in Alberta

Government Organization Act
c. G-10 Schedule 7.1

s. 2(1) The following, carried out in relation to or as part of providing a health service, are restricted activities:

(a)    to cut a body tissue, to administer anything by an invasive procedure on body tissue or to perform surgical or other invasive procedures on body tissue

(i)    below the dermis or the mucous membrane or in or below the surface of the cornea;

(ii)    in or below the surface of teeth, including scaling of teeth;

(b)    to insert or remove instruments, devices, fingers or hands

(i)    beyond the cartilaginous portion of the ear canal,

(ii)    beyond the point in the nasal passages where they normally narrow,

(iii)    beyond the pharynx,

(iv)    beyond the opening of the urethra,

(v)    beyond the labia majora,

(vi)    beyond the anal verge, or

(vii)    into an artificial opening into the body;

(b.1)    to insert into the ear canal

      (i)   under pressure, liquid, air or gas;

      (ii)   a substance that subsequently solidifies;

(c)   to set or reset a fracture of a bone;

(d)   to reduce a dislocation of a joint except for a partial dislocation of the joints of the fingers and toes;

(e)   to use a deliberate, brief, fast thrust to move the joints of the spine beyond the normal range but within the anatomical range of motion, which generally results in an audible click or pop;

(f)   to prescribe a Schedule 1 drug within the meaning of the *Pharmacy and Drug Act*;[14]

(g)   to dispense, compound, provide for selling or sell a Schedule 1 drug or Schedule 2 drug within the meaning of the *Pharmacy and Drug Act*;

(h)   to administer a vaccine or parenteral nutrition;

(i)   to prescribe, compound or administer blood or blood products;

(j)   to prescribe or administer diagnostic imaging contrast agents;

(k)   to prescribe or administer anesthetic gases, including nitrous oxide, for the purposes of anesthesia or sedation;

(l)   to prescribe or administer radiopharmaceuticals, radiolabelled substances, radioactive gases or radioaerosols;

(m)   to order or apply any form of ionizing radiation in

      (i)   medical radiography,

      (ii)   nuclear medicine, or

      (iii)   radiation therapy;

(n)   to order or apply non-ionizing radiation in

      (i)   lithotripsy,

      (ii)   magnetic resonance imaging, or

      (iii)   ultrasound imaging, including any application of ultrasound to a fetus;

(o)   to prescribe or fit

      (i)   an orthodontic or periodontal appliance,

      (ii)   a fixed or removable partial or complete denture, or

      (iii)   an implant supported prosthesis;

(p)   to perform a psychosocial intervention with an expectation of treating a substantial disorder of thought, mood, perception, orientation or memory that grossly impairs

---

[14] Schedule 1 and Schedule 2 drugs do not include Natural Health Products as defined by the *Natural Health Products Regulations* to the *Canada Food and Drugs Act*.

> (i)   judgment,
>
> (ii)   behaviour,
>
> (iii)   capacity to recognize reality, or
>
> (iv)   ability to meet the ordinary demands of life;

(q)   to manage labour or deliver a baby;

(r)   to prescribe or dispense corrective lenses.

s. 4(1) No person shall perform a restricted activity or a portion of it on or for another person unless

> (a) the person performing it
>
> > (i) is a regulated member as defined in the Health Professions Act, and is authorized to perform it by the regulations under the Health Professions Act,
> >
> > (ii) is authorized to perform it by a regulation under section 3,
> >
> > (ii.1) is authorized to perform it by an order under section 3.1, or
> >
> > (iii) is authorized to perform it by another enactment, or
>
> (b) the person performing it
>
> > (i) has the consent of, and is being supervised by, a regulated member described in clause (a)(i), and
> >
> > (ii) is permitted to perform the restricted activity under a regulation made under section 131(1)(d)(i) of the Health Professions Act by the council of the college of the regulated member referred to in subclause (i), and there are regulations made under section 131(1)(d)(ii) of the Health Professions Act by the council of the college of that regulated member respecting how regulated members must supervise persons who provide restricted activities under this clause.

s. 5(1) A person who contravenes section 4 is guilty of an offence and liable

(a) for a first offence, to a fine of not more than $5,000,

(b) for a 2nd offence, to a fine of not more than $10,000, and

(c) for a 3rd and every subsequent offence, to a fine of not more than $25,000 or to imprisonment for a term of not more than 6 months or to both fine and imprisonment.

Health Professions Act

c. H-7

s. 46(1) A person must apply for registration if the person

(a) meets the requirements of section 28(2) for registration as a regulated member, and

(b) intends to provide one or more of the following:

(i) professional services directly to the public;

## Restrictions on Professional Titles in Alberta

Health Professions Act
c. H-7

s. 128(1) No person or group of persons shall represent or imply that the person is a regulated member or that the group of persons consists of regulated members unless the person is a regulated member or the group of persons consists of regulated members.

(2)  No person or group of persons shall use the name of a college, alone or in combination with other words, in a manner that states or implies that the person or group of persons is a college under this Act unless the person or group of persons is a college under this Act.

(3)  No regulated member shall use the word "registered" in a manner that states or implies that the member is a regulated member of a regulated profession except in accordance with the regulations.

(4)  No person or group of persons shall use the word "regulated" in connection with the name of a regulated profession or professional service or the words "regulated health professional" in a manner that states or implies that the person or group of persons is a college or a regulated member or group of regulated members unless the person or group of persons is a college under this Act or another enactment or is a regulated member or consists of a group of regulated members.

(5)  No person other than

(a)    a regulated member shall use a title, abbreviation or initials set out in section 2 of a schedule to this Act alone or in combination with other words in a manner that states or implies that the person is a regulated member of the college to which section 2 of the schedule refers, or

(b)    a student who is enrolled in a program that in the opinion of the registrar is a program to train persons to provide professional services shall use a title, abbreviation or initials set out in section 2 of a schedule to this Act in combination with the word "student" while undertaking activities related to the program.

(10)    No person or group of persons shall use the word "registered" or "regulated" or the phrase "regulated health professional" alone or in combination with other words that in a manner states or implies that the person is a regulated member unless the person or group of persons

(a)  is a regulated member or consists of a group of regulated members, or

(b)  is a person or group of persons authorized to use the word "registered" or "regulated" or the phrase "regulated health professional" in connection with the health service by another enactment.

s. 129 A person who contravenes section 128 is guilty of an offence and liable

(a) for a first offence, to a fine of not more than $2,000,

(b) for a 2nd offence, to a fine of not more than $4,000, and

(c) for a 3rd and every subsequent offence, to a fine of not more than $6000 or to imprisonment for a term of not more than 6 months or to both fine and imprisonment. 1999 cH-5.5 s1

Health Professions Act
c. H-7, Schedule 23
Profession of Registered Dietitians and Registered Nutritionists

s. 2.   A regulated member of the College of Dietitians of Alberta may, as authorized by the regulations, use any of the following titles, abbreviations and initials:

(a)  registered dietitian;

(b)  dietitian;

(b.1) provisional dietitian;

(b.2) dietetic intern

(b.3) nutritionist

(c)  registered nutritionist

(d)  repealed

(e)  R.D.

## British Columbia

The provision of health services in British Columbia is regulated using a Restricted Activity framework. The rules that impact the practices of Holistic Nutritionists are primarily found in the *Health Professions Act*, and the regulations under this Act: *Medical Practitioners Regulation, Naturopathic Physicians Regulation*, the *Dietitians Regulation and the Chinese Medical Practitioners Regulation*. Under section 4 of the B.C. *Offence Act*[15] a breach of the *Health Professions Act* and its regulations can result in a fine of up to $2,000, and/or imprisonment for a term of up to six months.

Unlike other provinces that regulate using the Restricted Activity framework, as this is being written, B.C. has not yet published a complete list of Restricted Activities in one place. (The most recent draft of the proposed Restricted Activities was published for discussion in March 2010 and is included in the legislative summaries at the end of this section.) Rather, activities that are restricted to members of a specific Regulated Health Profession and any other activities its members are authorized to perform are set out in the regulation that creates that Regulated Health Profession. For example, section 5 of the *Dietitians Regulation* provides that, "No person other than a registrant who meets the additional qualifications set out in the bylaws of the college may (a) design, compound or dispense therapeutic diets if nutrition is administered through enteral means, (b) design therapeutic diets if nutrition is administered through parenteral means, or (c) administer a substance to a person by instillation through enteral or parenteral means." Subsection 13(2) of the *Health Professions Act* prohibits any person other than an authorized registrant of a college from providing a service (i.e., a Restricted Activity) that is reserved to members of that college unless another exemption exists. For example, under the *Medical Practitioners Regulation* physicians are authorized to perform any restricted activity.

The approach used by B.C. makes it more difficult than in other provinces for the public to know exactly what activities are restricted.

The *Medical Practitioners Regulation* does not contain a list of Restricted Activities. Rather it defines certain broad activities to be medical services, then prohibits anyone other than a physician from providing a service if that service was previously restricted under the old *Medical Practitioners Act* (which was otherwise repealed by the *Health Professions Act*). Services of medicine are defined to include, among other things, the assessment and

---

[15] *Offence Act* [RSBC 1996] Chapter 338

management of a physical or mental condition, the prevention and treatment of physical and mental diseases and the promotion of good health.

The good news for Holistic Nutritionists is that the old *Medical Practitioners Act* restricted only the practice of traditional areas of medicine, such as diagnosing and prescribing treatments for diseases and disorders, and did not restrict activities such as disease prevention and the promotion of good health. So while Holistic Nutritionists are still prohibited from diagnosing and treating diseases and disorders in B.C., they are not currently prohibited from assisting clients to prevent disease or improve health.

The regulatory approach currently in place in B.C. relating to the practice of medicine is somewhat of a hybrid model because it partly regulates through a definition of medicine (which is the Professional Exclusivity approach) as well through a list Restricted Activities. Since the activity of treating diseases or disorders is not included in the consolidated draft list of Restricted Activities, but continues to be a restricted medical service under this dual approach, we will have to wait to see if Holistic Nutritionists become free to provide treatments, if and when a complete list of Restricted Activities formally becomes part of the regulations and if this legacy from the old *Medical Practitioners Act* is rescinded.

Section 5 of the *Naturopathic Physicians Regulation* restricts the practice of naturopathic medicine to registered naturopaths. Naturopathic medicine is defined to be providing the services of: "prevention, assessment and treatment of an individual's diseases, disorders and conditions using education and naturopathic techniques, therapies or therapeutics to stimulate or support healing processes and promote, maintain or restore the overall health of the individual." The Regulation does reserve any Restricted Activities for the exclusive practice of naturopaths, and, therefore, does not restrict the services that can be provided by a conventional Holistic Nutritionist.

The *Dietitians Regulation* defines the scope of a registered a dietitian's practice. Section 5 of the Regulation defines and reserves several Restricted Activities that may only be performed by qualified registered dietitians. As cited earlier, these include designing therapeutic diets that are to be administered by enteral or parenteral means, compounding and dispensing diets that are to be administered by enteral means, and administering substances by instillation through enteral or parenteral means.

The *Dietitians Regulation* reserves the title "Dietitian" for the exclusive use of registered dietitians. As neither the Act nor the Regulation restrict in any way the use of the title "Nutritionist," use of this title in B.C. is not restricted.

In British Columbia, it is also relevant to consider the *Traditional Chinese Medicine Practitioners and Acupuncturists Regulation* as it includes a restriction relating to the prescription of herbal remedies, which a Holistic Nutritionist could accidentally breach. Section 5 of this Regulation provides that only a traditional Chinese medicine practitioner or a herbalist (which is another category of registrant under the Regulation) may "prescribe those Chinese herbal formulae listed in a schedule to the bylaws of the College." The College's bylaws available on-line do not currently include a list of restricted formulae. My calls to the College to confirm this state of affairs went unanswered. A Holistic Nutritionist who prescribes Chinese herbal remedies as part of his or her practice must contact the College periodically to ensure they comply with this restriction.

At the present time, a Holistic Nutritionist who is not a member of a Regulated Health Profession in B.C. may carry on a conventional nutritional practice provided he or she: (1) does not provide a restricted service of "medicine" (such as diagnosing and treating diseases and disorders) as this term is defined in the *Medical Practitioners Regulation*; (2) does not perform a Restricted Activity described in the *Dietitians Regulation* or any of the other regulations under the *Health Professions Act*, (3) does not prescribe Chinese herbal remedies which are contained on a restricted list maintained by the College of Traditional Chinese Medicine Practitioners and Acupuncturists of British Columbia, (4) does not market themselves to the public using a title reserved for registered dietitians or any another Regulated Health Profession or otherwise falsely represent themselves as being a member of a Regulated Health Profession; and (5) otherwise complies with laws of general application.

For a better understanding of how terms such as "diagnose" and "treat," etc. are to be interpreted, the reader should review the discussion of terminology in the next chapter.

### Restrictions on Activities in British Columbia

The Medical Practitioners Regulation
B.C. Reg. 416/2008

s.1 In this regulation:

"medicine" means the health profession in which a person provides the services of

>   (a) assessment and management of the physical or mental condition of an individual or group of individuals at any stage of the biological life cycle, including the prenatal and postmortem periods,

>   (b) prevention and treatment of physical and mental diseases, disorders and conditions, and

(c) promotion of good health;

s. 4 (1) A registrant in the course of practising medicine may perform any restricted activity.

(2) Only a registrant may provide a service of medicine as set out in this regulation if, on the day before this section comes into force, the provision of the same service by anyone other than a person authorized under the Medical Practitioners Act was prohibited.

The Dietitians Regulation
B.C. Reg. 279/2008

s. 1 In this regulation:

"Act" means the Health Professions Act;

"compound" means to mix ingredients for parenteral or enteral nutrition;

"dietetics" means the assessment of nutritional needs, design, implementation and evaluation of nutritional care plans and therapeutic diets, the science of food and human nutrition, and dissemination of information about food and human nutrition to attain, maintain and promote the health of individuals, groups and the community;

"design" means the selection of appropriate ingredients for parenteral or enteral nutrition;

"dispense" means to fill a prescription for parenteral or enteral nutrition;

"enteral" means administration of a nutritional substance to a patient by means of a feeding tube into the gastrointestinal tract;

"parenteral" means administration of a nutritional substance to a patient directly into the blood stream.

Restricted activities

s.5 No person other than a registrant who meets the additional qualifications set out in the bylaws of the college may

   (a) design, compound or dispense therapeutic diets if nutrition is administered through enteral means,

   (b) design therapeutic diets if nutrition is administered through parenteral means, or

   (c) administer a substance to a person by instillation through enteral or parenteral means.

Traditional Chinese Medicine Practitioners
and Acupuncturist Regulation
B.C. Reg. 290/2008

s. 1 In this regulation:

"doctor of traditional Chinese medicine" means a traditional Chinese medicine practitioner who is authorized under the bylaws to use the title "doctor of traditional Chinese medicine";

"herbalist" means a registrant authorized under the bylaws to prescribe, compound or dispense Chinese herbal formulae (Zhong Yao Chu Fang) and Chinese food cure recipes (Shi Liao);

"prescribe" means to give directions, either orally or in writing, for the preparation and administration of a traditional Chinese medicine remedy to be used in the treatment of a disorder or an imbalance;

"traditional Chinese medicine" means the promotion, maintenance and restoration of health and prevention of a disorder, imbalance or disease based on traditional Chinese medicine theory by utilization of the primary therapies of

> (a) Chinese acupuncture (Zhen), moxibustion (Jiu) and suction cup (Ba Guan),
>
> (b) Chinese manipulative therapy (Tui Na),
>
> (c) Chinese energy control therapy (Qi Gong),
>
> (d) Chinese rehabilitation exercises such as Chinese shadow boxing (Tai Ji Quan), and
>
> (e) prescribing, compounding or dispensing Chinese herbal formulae (Zhong Yao Chu Fang) and Chinese food cure recipes (Shi Liao);

s. 5  No person other than a

> (a) traditional Chinese medicine practitioner, acupuncturist or herbalist may make a traditional Chinese medicine diagnosis identifying a disease, disorder or condition as the cause of signs or symptoms,
>
> (b) traditional Chinese medicine practitioner or a herbalist may prescribe those Chinese herbal formulae listed in a schedule to the bylaws of the College, and
>
> (c) traditional Chinese medicine practitioner or an acupuncturist may insert acupuncture needles under the skin for the purposes of practising acupuncture.

Health Professions Act
RSBC 1996 C. 183

s. 13 (1) If a regulation under section 12 (2) (d) limits the services that may be provided in the course of practice of a designated health profession, a registrant must limit his or her practice of that designated health profession in accordance with the regulation.

(2) If a regulation under section 12 (2) (e) prescribes a service that may only be provided by a registrant of a particular college,

> (a) a person other than a registrant of the college must not provide the service, and
>
> (b) a person must not recover any fee or remuneration in any court in respect of the provision of the service unless, at the time the service was provided, the person was

a registrant of the college or a corporation entitled to provide the services of a registrant of the college.

### Proposed List of Restricted Activities, March 2010
*Current draft of proposed Restricted Activities*

1. Making a diagnosis identifying a disease, disorder or condition as the cause of signs or symptoms of the individual.

2. Performing the following physically invasive or physically manipulative acts:

   a. procedures on tissue below the dermis, below the surface of a mucous membrane, in or below the surface of the cornea, in or below the surfaces of the teeth, including the scaling of teeth;

   b. setting or casting a fracture of a bone or reducing a dislocation of a joint;

   c. movement of the joints of the spine beyond the limits the body can voluntarily achieve but within the anatomical range of motion using a high velocity, low amplitude thrust;

   d. administering a substance, other than a drug,

      i. by injection,

      ii. by inhalation,

      iii. by mechanical ventilation

      iv. by irrigation, or

      v. by instillation through enteral or parenteral means; and

   e. putting an instrument, hand or finger(s),

      i. into the external ear canal, including applying pressurized air or water,

      ii. beyond the point in the nasal passages, where they normally narrow,

      iii. beyond the pharynx,

      iv. beyond the opening of the urethra,

      v. beyond the labia majora,

      vi. beyond the anal verge, or

      vii. into an artificial opening into the body.

3. Managing labour or delivery of a baby.

4. Applying or ordering the application of a hazardous form of energy including diagnostic ultrasound, electricity, magnetic resonance imaging, lithotripsy, laser and X-ray, or as prescribed by regulation.

5.

   a. Prescribing, compounding, dispensing or administering by any means a drug listed in Schedule I or II of the Pharmacists, Pharmacy Operations and Drug Scheduling Act.

For the purposes of this reserved act, the following definitions shall apply:

"prescribing": the ordering of a drug.

"compounding": mixing ingredients, at least one of which is a drug.

"dispensing": preparing or filling a prescription for drugs.

b. Designing, compounding or dispensing therapeutic diets where nutrition is administered through enteral or parenteral means.

For the purposes of this reserved act, the following definitions shall apply:

"designing": the selection of appropriate ingredients for enteral or parenteral nutrition.

"compounding": mixing ingredients, for enteral or parenteral nutrition

"dispensing": filling a prescription for enteral or parenteral nutrition.

6. Prescribing appliances or devices for vision, hearing or dental conditions; dispensing such prescribed appliances or devices for dental conditions; fitting such appliances or devices for dental conditions, or fitting contact lenses.

For the purposes of this reserved act, the following definitions shall apply:

"prescribing": ordering the fabrication or alteration of appliances or devices for vision, hearing, or dental conditions.

"dispensing": filling a prescription by fabricating or altering a dental appliance or device.

a. Allergy challenge testing or allergy desensitizing treatment involving injection, scratch tests or inhalation, and allergy challenge testing by any means with respect to a patient who has had a previous anaphylactic reaction;

b. Cardiac stress testing conducted for medical diagnosis and treatment planning.

## Restrictions on Professional Titles in British Columbia

Dietitians Regulation
B.C. Reg. 279/2008

s. 3 The title "dietitian" is reserved for exclusive use by registrants

Health Professions Act
RSBC 1996 C. 183

s.12.1 (1) If a regulation under section 12 (2) (b) prescribes a title to be used exclusively by registrants of a college, a person other than a registrant of the college must not use the title, an abbreviation of the title or an equivalent of the title or abbreviation in another language

    (a) to describe the person's work,

    (b) in association with or as part of another title describing the person's work, or

    (c) in association with a description of the person's work.

(2) If a regulation under section 12 (2) (b.1) prescribes a limit or condition respecting the use of a title, the title must not be used except in accordance with the regulation.

(3) A person other than a registrant of a college must not use a name, title, description or abbreviation of a name or title, or an equivalent of a name or title in another language, in any manner that expresses or implies that he or she is a registrant or associated with the college.

## Manitoba

As this is being written, the province of Manitoba is in the process of making the transition to a Restricted Activities framework (called "Reserved Acts" in Manitoba) under *The Regulated Health Professions Act* which was proclaimed into force on December 20, 2013. By June 2015 two professions, audiologists and speech-language pathologists, had completed the transition to the new framework and physicians, dietitians or naturopaths, among others, were still working towards this goal. During the transition period the Act grants registered members of all Manitoba Regulated Health Professions an exemption from the Reserved Acts, provided services are performed in compliance with the rules of their regulatory college and enabling legislation. The public must comply with the Reserved Acts. The unlawful practice of a Reserved Act by an individual can result in a fine of up to $10,000 for a first offence.

Until physicians, dietitians and naturopaths make their transition to regulation under *The Regulated Health Professions Act*, Holistic Nutritionists in Manitoba must continue to refer to and comply with *The Medical Act, The Naturopathic Act* and *The Registered Dietitians Act*, as well as *The Regulated Health Professions Act*. The list of Reserved Acts is set out at the end of this section.

Section 66 of *The Medical Act* makes it an offence to practice medicine or to hold yourself out as being qualified to practice medicine unless licensed to do so under the Act. Section 2 of *The Medical Act* sets out certain activities, the practice of which is deemed to be the practice of medicine. These include, among other things, diagnosing and treating diseases and disorders. This is not an exhaustive list, however, so the question of whether in providing services a Holistic Nutritionist is practising medicine will, for the time being, also be determined by the courts. Under *The Medical Act* the unlawful practice of medicine can result in a fine of up to $6,000 for a first offence.

Once the regulation of physicians is transitioned to *The Regulated Health Professions Act, The Medical Act* rescinded, and the practice of medicine restrictions contained within it removed, Holistic Nutritionists will gain the ability to treat (but not diagnose) diseases and disorders as the provision of a treatment is not in and of itself a Reserved Act (i.e., it is not prohibited unless the type of treatment involves a specific activity that is on the list).

*The Naturopathic Act* makes it an offence to practice naturopathy or use the title "Naturopath" unless authorized to do so under the Act. *The Naturopathic Act* also defines the practice of naturopathy to be "a drugless system of therapy that treats human injuries, ailments, or diseases, by natural methods." Since the treatment of "injuries, ailments, or diseases" etc. by any method is already restricted by *The Medical Act*, this restriction in *The Naturopathic Act* does not further limit the area of practice that is presently open to Holistic Nutritionists in Manitoba. As with *The Medical Act* this restriction will be removed once the regulation of naturopaths is transitioned to *The Regulated Health Professions Act* and *The Naturopathic Act* rescinded.

*The Registered Dietitians Act* defines the scope of a registered dietitian's practice. While it does not restrict an unregulated professional from carrying on a dietitian's practice, it does make it unlawful to wrongfully imply you are a registered dietitian entitled to engage in the practice of dietetics.

Sections 77 to 81 of *The Regulated Health Professions Act* regulates the use of professional titles in Manitoba. Section 77 is a general prohibition against using a title that wrongly implies you are a member of a Regulated Health Profession. Section 81 is a general prohibition against using "registered" or "licensed" as part of a title, unless you are a member of a Regulated Health Profession whose college provides such a service, or you are otherwise permitted to do so under the Act's regulations. The way *The Regulated Health Professions Act* is structured, it appears the granting of specific titles such as "Dietitian," will continue to primarily take place in the enabling legislation for each Regulated Health Profession. As noted earlier, a breach of *The Regulated Health Professions Act* by an individual can result in a fine of up to $10,000 for a first offence.

At the present time *The Registered Dietitians Act* reserves the title "Dietitian" and several related variations for the exclusive use of registered dietitians. As the Act does not restrict in any way the use of the title "Nutritionist," Holistic Nutritionists may use this word as part of a professional title or in their advertising and marketing materials. A breach of *The Registered Dietitians Act* can result in a fine of up to $10,000.Holistic Nutritionists in Manitoba will have to watch for changes when the regulation of dietitians is transitioned to *The Regulated Health Professions Act* and a new *Dietitians Act* is put in place.

As this is being written a Holistic Nutritionist who is not a member of a Regulated Health Profession in Manitoba may carry on a conventional nutritional practice provided he or she: (1) does not "practice medicine" as this term is defined in *The Medical Act* and has been interpreted by the courts (until such time as the regulation of physicians is transitioned to *The Regulated Health Professions Act*, after which this restriction will cease to apply); (2) does not practice naturopathy as defined in the *Naturopathic Act* (until such time as the regulation of naturopaths is transitioned to the *Regulated Health Professions Act*, after which this restriction will cease to apply); (3) does not perform a Reserved Act under *The Regulated Health Professions Act;* (4) does not market themselves to the public using a title reserved for registered dietitians or any another Regulated Health Profession, that otherwise infers they are a member of a Regulated Health Profession, or that uses the words 'registered' or 'licensed'; and (5) otherwise complies with laws of general application.

For a better understanding of how terms such as "practice of medicine," "diagnose" and "treat," etc. are to be interpreted, the reader should review the discussion of terminology in the next chapter.

### Restrictions on Activities in Manitoba

The Regulated Health Professions Act
S.M. 2009, c. 15

s. 4    A "reserved act" is any of the following acts done with respect to an individual in the course of providing health care:

1. Making a diagnosis and communicating it to an individual or his or her personal representative in circumstances in which it is reasonably foreseeable that the individual or representative will rely on the diagnosis to make a decision about the individual's health care.

2. Ordering or receiving reports of screening or diagnostic tests.

3. Performing a procedure on tissue

   (a) below the dermis;

   (b) below the surface of a mucous membrane;

   (c) on or below the surface of the cornea; or

   (d) on or below the surface of a tooth or dental implant, including the scaling of a tooth or dental implant.

4. Inserting or removing an instrument or a device, hand or finger

   (a) into the external ear canal;

   (b) beyond the point in the nasal passages where they normally narrow;

   (c) beyond the pharynx;

   (d) beyond the opening of the urethra;

   (e) beyond the labia majora;

   (f) beyond the anal verge; or

   (g) into an artificial opening in the body.

5. Administering a substance

   (a) by injection;

(b) by inhalation;

(c) by mechanical ventilation;

(d) by irrigation;

(e) by enteral instillation or parenteral instillation;

(f) by transfusion; or

(g) using a hyperbaric chamber.

6. Prescribing a drug or vaccine.

7. Compounding a drug or vaccine.

8. Dispensing or selling a drug or vaccine.

9. Administering a drug or vaccine by any method.

10. Applying or ordering the application of

(a) ultrasound for diagnostic or imaging purposes, including any application of ultrasound to a fetus;

(b) electricity for

(i) aversive conditioning,

(ii) cardiac pacemaker therapy,

(iii) cardioversion,

(iv) defibrillation,

(v) electrocoagulation,

(vi) electroconvulsive shock therapy,

(vii) electromyography,

(viii) fulguration,

(ix) nerve conduction studies, or

(x) transcutaneous cardiac pacing;

(c) electromagnetism for magnetic resonance imaging;

(d) other non-ionizing radiation for the purpose of cutting or destroying tissue or medical imagery;

(e) X-rays or other ionizing radiation for diagnostic, imaging or therapeutic purposes, including computerized axial tomography, positron emission tomography and radiation therapy;

(f) any other use of a form of energy listed in clauses (a) to (e), if the use is specified by regulation; or

(g) any other form of energy that is specified by regulation.

11. In relation to a therapeutic diet that is administered by enteral instillation or parenteral instillation,

(a) selecting ingredients for the diet; or

(b) compounding or administering the diet.

12. Setting or casting a fracture of a bone or a dislocation of a joint.

13. Putting into the external ear canal, up to the eardrum, a substance that

(a) is under pressure; or

(b) subsequently solidifies.

14. Managing labour or the delivery of a baby.

15. Administering a high velocity, low amplitude thrust to move a joint of the spine within its anatomical range of motion.

16. Prescribing, dispensing or fitting a wearable hearing instrument.

17. Prescribing, dispensing or verifying a vision appliance.

18. Fitting a contact lens.

19. Prescribing, dispensing or fitting a dental appliance.

20. Performing a psycho-social intervention with an expectation of modifying a substantial disorder of thought, mood, perception, orientation or memory that grossly impairs judgment, behaviour, the capacity to recognize reality, or the ability to meet the ordinary demands of life.

21. In relation to allergies,

(a) performing challenge testing by any method; or

(b) performing desensitizing treatment by any method.

s. 171(1) A person who contravenes a provision of this Act, other than section 140 (confidentiality of information), or of the regulations is guilty of an offence and is liable on summary conviction to a fine

(a) in the case of an individual,

(i) for a first offence, to a fine of not more than $10,000, and

(ii) for each subsequent offence, to a fine of not more than $50,000; and

(b) in the case of a corporation,

(i) for a first offence, to a fine of not more than $25,000, and

(ii) for each subsequent offence, to a fine of not more than $100,000.

## The Medical Act
## C.C.S.M. c. M90
*(To be rescinded on a date yet to be determined)*

s. 2(1)  Without restricting the generality of the definition of practice of medicine, a person shall be deemed to be practising medicine within the meaning of this Act who

(a) by advertisement, sign, or statement of any kind, written or oral, alleges or implies or states that he is, or holds himself out as being, qualified, able, or willing, to diagnose, prescribe for, prevent, or treat, any human disease, ailment, deformity, defect, or injury, or to perform any operation or surgery to remedy any human disease, ailment, deformity, defect, or injury, or to examine or advise upon the physical or mental condition of any person; or

(b) diagnoses, or offers to diagnose, or attempts by any means whatsoever to diagnose, any human disease, ailment, deformity, defect, or injury, or who examines or advises upon, or offers to examine or advise upon, the physical or mental condition of any person; or

(c) prescribes or administers any drugs, serum, medicine, or any substance or remedy, whether for the cure, treatment, or prevention, of any human disease, ailment, deformity, defect, or injury; or

(d) prescribes or administers any treatment, or performs any operation or manipulation, or applies any apparatus or appliance, for the cure, treatment, or prevention, of any human disease, ailment, deformity, defect, or injury, or acts as a midwife; or

(e) repealed, S.M. 1999, c. 39, s. 3.

s. 66(2)  Any person not licensed under this Act who practices or professes to practice medicine in the province, is guilty of an offence.

s. 68.1  A person who is guilty of an offence under this Act is liable, on summary conviction,

(a) for a first offence, to a fine of not more than $6,000; and

(b) for a second or subsequent offence, to a fine of not more than $30,000.

## The Registered Dietitians Act,
## C.C.S.M. c. R39
*(To be rescinded on a date yet to be determined)*

s. 2  The practice of dietetics means the translation and application of scientific knowledge of food and human nutrition through

(a) assessment, design, implementation and evaluation of nutritional interventions;

(b) integration of food and nutrition principles in the management of food service systems; and

(c) dissemination of information to attain, maintain, promote and protect the health of individuals, groups and the community.

Representation as a registered dietitian or dietitian

s. 3(1)   No person except a registered dietitian shall

(a) represent or hold out, expressly or by implication, that he or she is a registered dietitian or a dietitian, or is entitled to engage in the practice of dietetics as a registered dietitian or as a dietitian; or

(b) use any sign, display, title or advertisement implying that he or she is a registered dietitian or a dietitian.

s. 58(1)   A person who contravenes a provision of this Act or the regulations, other than section 62 of this Act, is guilty of an offence and is liable on summary conviction to a fine of not more than $10,000.

## Restriction on Professional Titles in Manitoba

The Regulated Health Professions Act
S.M. 2009, c. 15

s. 77   No person shall use a name, title, description or abbreviation in a manner that expresses or implies that he or she is a member of a college, unless the person is a member of that college.

s. 78(1)   No person shall use the title "doctor," surgeon" or "physician" — or a variation or abbreviation of any of them or an equivalent in another language — in the course of providing health care unless the person is permitted to use the title, variation or abbreviation by this Act or another Act.

s. 81(1)   No person who is providing health care shall use the term "registered" or "licensed," or a variation or abbreviation of either of them or an equivalent in another language, in association with or as part of the title describing his or her work, unless that person

(a) is a member of a college whose members provide that type of health care; and

(b) is using that term in accordance with the regulations.

s. 81(2)   Despite subsection (1) but subject to section 77, a person may use the term "registered" or "licensed" as part of a title describing his or her work if

(a) the person is a member of an organization or class of organizations specified by regulation; or

(b) the person is authorized in another jurisdiction to use the title to indicate membership in a body substantially similar to the college in Manitoba that regulates that health profession and, in using the title, indicates

(i) the name of the other jurisdiction, and

(ii) that he or she is currently authorized to practice the health profession in the other jurisdiction.

## The Registered Dietitians Act
### C.C.S.M. c. R39

s. 3(2) No person except a registered dietitian shall use the title "registered dietitian" or "dietitian", a variation or abbreviation of either title, or an equivalent of either title in another language.

Use of title "graduate dietitian"

s. 3(3) Unless authorized by the council, no person except a graduate dietitian shall use the title "graduate dietitian", a variation or abbreviation of that title, or an equivalent in another language.

Use of title "dietetic intern"

s. 3(4) Unless authorized by the council, no person except a person enrolled in a dietetic education program referred to in subclause 9(2)(a)(i) shall use the title "dietetic intern", a variation or abbreviation of that title, or an equivalent in another.

s. 58(1)  A person who contravenes a provision of this Act or the regulations, other than section 62 of this Act, is guilty of an offence and is liable on summary conviction to a fine of not more than $10,000.

## New Brunswick

The provision of health services in New Brunswick is regulated using a Professional Exclusivity framework. The rules that impact the practices of Holistic Nutritionists are primarily found in the *Medical Act* and *An Act Respecting the New Brunswick Association of Dietitians* (the *"Dietitians Act"*). Naturopathy is not a regulated profession in New Brunswick.

Section 43 of the *Medical Act* makes it an offence to practice or hold yourself out to be able to practice medicine, unless licensed to do so under the Act. Section 3 of the *Medical Act* provides an illustrative list of practice areas (medicine, surgery, and osteopathic medicine and the specialties and subspecialties thereof) that are deemed to be included within the meaning of "medicine." As the definition of the practice of medicine in the Act does not include any defined activities, the question of whether in providing services a Holistic Nutritionist is practising medicine would be determined by the courts, although practising medicine is generally interpreted to include, among other things, diagnosing and treating diseases and disorders. A breach of the *Medical Act* can result in a fine of up to $10,000, and/or imprisonment for a term of up to six months.

Section 2 of the *Dietitians Act* expansively defines the practice area of a registered dietitian and section 12 prohibits unregistered persons from providing such services to the public. For example, this Act defines the practice of dietetics to mean "the translation and application of the scientific knowledge of food and human nutrition towards the attainment, maintenance and promotion of the health of individuals" and includes within this "assessing nutritional needs of individuals and developing and implementing nutritional care plans based on the assessments" and "establishing and reviewing the principles of nutrition and guidelines for healthy and ill people throughout their lives." Unless you are a registered dietitian (or a member of another Regulated Health Profession whose practice area includes nutritional counselling, such as a physician) not only must you avoid treating diseases and disorders nutritionally, you must avoid the business of performing assessments and providing advice to individuals that promotes wellness.

Section 12 of the *Dietitians Act* also reserves the titles "Dietitian" and "Registered Dietitian-Nutritionist," among others, for exclusive use by registered dietitians. As the Act does not reserve use of the word "Nutritionist" on its own, it may be used on its own or in combination with other words (other than as part of the phrase "Registered Dietitian—Nutritionist") in marketing literature. However, since the Act also restricts the use of other designations that "represent" the restricted title, the use of "Nutritionist" as part of a professional title should be avoided.

A breach of the *Dietitians Act* can result in a fine of up to $2,000, and/or imprisonment.

As a result of the rules contained in the *Medical Act* and the *Dietitians Act,* I do not believe it is possible for a Holistic Nutritionist to lawfully carry on a conventional nutritional counselling practice in the province of New Brunswick.

For a better understanding of how terms such as "practice of medicine" are to be interpreted, the reader should review the discussion of terminology in the next chapter.

### Restrictions on Activities in New Brunswick

The Medical Act, 1981

s. 3 "practice of medicine" includes the practice of medicine, surgery, and osteopathic medicine and the specialties and subspecialties thereof;

s. 43(2) A person who practices medicine

(a) while his licence is suspended or revoked, or

(b) without a licence,

commits an offence.

s. 45(1) Except as provided in this Act and the regulations, no person, other than a medical practitioner who holds a licence or a professional corporation which holds a licence shall

(a) publicly or privately, for hire, gain or hope of reward, practice or offer to practice medicine;

(b) hold himself out in any way to be entitled to practice medicine; or

(c) use any title or description implying or designed to lead the public to believe that he is entitled to practice medicine.

s. 50(1) A person who violates

(a) any provision of this Act,

(b) any provision of a regulation enacted under paragraphs 7(2) (q), (r), (s), or

(c) any provision of a regulation enacted under paragraphs 30(2)(e), 31(2)(a), or 31(2)(c)

commits an offence and is liable on summary conviction to a fine not exceeding ten thousand dollars, or to imprisonment for a term not exceeding six months, or to both.

An Act Respecting the New Brunswick Association of Dietitians
C. 75 1988

s. 2 "practice of dietetics" means the translation and application of the scientific knowledge of foods and human nutrition towards the attainment, maintenance and promotion of the health of individuals, groups and the community and includes the following:

(a) administering food service systems though this function is not exclusive to dietitians;

(b) assessing nutritional needs of individuals and developing and implementing nutritional care plans based on the assessments;

(c) establishing and reviewing the principles of nutrition and guidelines for healthy and ill people throughout their lives;

(d) assessing the overall nutritional needs of a community in order to establish priorities and to influence  policies which provide the nutritional  component of preventative programs, and implementing and evaluating those programs;

(e)  interpreting and evaluating, for consumer protection, information on nutrition that is available to the public;

(f)  consulting with individuals, families and groups on the principles of food and nutrition and the practical application of those principles;

(g)  planning, conducting and evaluating educational programs on nutrition;

(h)  conducting basic and applied research in food, nutrition  and food service systems though this function is not exclusive to dietitians;

"registered dietitian" means a person who holds an annual certificate as a registered dietitian under this Act;

12(2) Except as provided in this Act, the by-laws or regulations no person shall engage in or hold herself out as engaging in the practice of dietetics unless she is registered under this Act.

s. 32 Any person who violates any provision of this Act, commits an offence and is liable on summary conviction to a fine not exceeding two thousand dollars, or to imprisonment, or both.

## Restrictions on Professional Titles in New Brunswick

An Act Respecting the New Brunswick Association of Dietitians
C. 75 1988

12(3) Except as provided in this Act, the by-laws or regulations no person shall use the title "Dietitian", "Dietician", "Professional Dietitian", "Registered Dietitian - Nutritionist", "Registered Dietitian", or the abbreviations "P.Dt.", "R.D." or "RON" or other designation representing the title, unless such person is a registered dietitian.

## Newfoundland and Labrador

The provision of health services in Newfoundland and Labrador is regulated using the Professional Exclusivity framework. The rules that impact the practices of Holistic Nutritionists are primarily found in the *Medical Act, 2011* and the *Dietitians Act*. Naturopathy is not a regulated profession in Newfoundland and Labrador.

Section 79 of the *Medical Act, 2011* makes it an offence to practice or to hold yourself out as being qualified to practice medicine, unless licensed to do so under the Act. Section 2 of the *Medical Ac*t contains an illustrative list of practice areas (e.g., cardiology, dermatology) that are deemed to be included within the meaning of practice of medicine. As the definition of the practice of medicine does not include any defined activities (apart from the practice of surgery on the human body) the question of whether in providing services a Holistic Nutritionist is practising medicine would be determined by the courts, although practising medicine is generally interpreted to include, among other things, diagnosing and treating diseases and disorders. A breach of the *Medical Act, 2011* can result in a fine of up to $10,000, and/or imprisonment for a term of up to six months.

The *Dietitians Act* does not define the practice of dietetics or grant exclusive rights to practice to registered dietitians. As a result, the Act does not restrict the practice of a Holistic Nutritionist. The *Dietitians Act* does, however, reserve the title "Dietitian" and several related variations for the exclusive use of registered dietitians. It also prohibits anyone who is not a registered dietitian from implying he or she is a registered dietitian. As the Act does not restrict in any way the use of the title "Nutritionist" Holistic Nutritionists may use this word as part of a professional title and in their marketing literature. A breach of the *Dietitians Act*, can result in a fine of up to $5,000, and/or imprisonment for a term of up to three months.

In addition to the legislation discussed above, Newfoundland and Labrador has implemented the *Health Professions Act* with a goal of establishing a more standardized regulatory approach to certain Regulated Health Professions. As this legislation does not amend the *Medical Act, 2011* or the *Dietitians Act*, it is not of immediate interest to Holistic Nutritionists, and therefore, is not summarized.

A Holistic Nutritionist who is not a member of a Regulated Health Profession in Newfoundland and Labrador may carry on a conventional nutritional practice provided he or she: (1) does not practice medicine as this term is defined in the *Medical Act, 2011* and defined by the courts; (2) does not market themselves to the public using a title reserved for registered dietitians, or any another Regulated Health Profession, or otherwise falsely represent themselves as being a member of a Regulated Health Profession; and (3) otherwise complies with laws of general application.

For a better understanding of how terms such as "practice of medicine" are to be interpreted, the reader should review the discussion of terminology in the next chapter.

## Restrictions on Activities in Newfoundland and Labrador

### Medical Act, 2011
### SNL 2011 c. M-4.02

s. 2. In this Act

(m) "practice of medicine" means the practice of medicine or surgery on the human body, and includes cardiology, dermatology, geriatrics, gynecology, neurology, obstetrics, ophthalmology, orthopedics, pathology, pediatrics, psychiatry and radiology and other specialities and subspecialties of medicine;

Offence

s. 79. (1) A person, other than a person who is licensed under this Act, shall not

   (a) engage in the practice of medicine;

   (b) hold himself or herself out or allege by advertisement, sign or statement of any kind to be entitled to engage in the practice of medicine; or

   (c) take or use a name, title or description implying or calculated to lead the public to believe that he or she is licensed under this Act.

(2) A person who violates subsection (1) is guilty of an offence and is liable upon summary conviction to a fine not exceeding $10,000 or to imprisonment for a term not exceeding 6 months or to both a fine and imprisonment.

(3) In a prosecution under this section, the onus of proof that the person accused of the offence has the right or privilege to engage in the practice of medicine is on the person accused.

## Restrictions on Professional Titles in Newfoundland and Labrador

### Dietitians Act
### SNL 2005 c. D-23.1

s. 20. (1) A person who is not a registered dietitian shall not take or use the titles "Dietitian" or "Registered Dietitian" or the initials "R.D." either alone or in combination with other words, letters or description that implies that the person is registered under this Act, or is entitled to be registered under this Act, or is recognized by law as a registered dietitian.

(2)   A person who contravenes this section is guilty of an offence and liable on summary conviction to a fine not exceeding $5,000 and in default of payment to imprisonment for a term not exceeding 3 months or to both a fine and imprisonment.

## Nova Scotia

The provision of health services in Nova Scotia is regulated using a Professional Exclusivity framework. The rules that impact the practices of Holistic Nutritionists are primarily found in the *Medical Act, Naturopathic Doctors Act* and *Professional Dietitians Act*.

A new *Medical Act* came into force in Nova Scotia in January 2015. Section 22 of this Act makes it an offence to practice medicine or to hold yourself out as being qualified to practice medicine unless licensed to do so under the Act. A major change introduced by this new Act is the definition of the practice of medicine. The new definition is extremely broad and includes "practices and procedures usually performed by a medical practitioner" including (i.e., not limited to) "the art and science of the assessment, diagnosis or treatment of an individual" and "the related promotion of health and the prevention of illness", and other practices and procedures taught in approved universities and schools.

This definition creates considerable uncertainty for Holistic Nutritionists.[16] To be characterized as the practice of medicine, activities must be within the scope of "practices and procedures usually performed by a medical practitioner." This core part of the definition is broad enough to include virtually any health related activity, while providing no detail or guidance. For example, many physicians make recommendations about improving diet and perhaps even taking nutritional supplements. Does this mean Holistic Nutritionists may not? Also note that the reference to diagnosing and treating individuals is not restricted to diagnosing or treating diseases and disorders, as is the case in most other provinces. This may mean that providing treatments unrelated to illness, to boost health and wellness for example, is now within the scope of the practice of medicine. The reference to "promotion of health and the prevention of illness" is also problematic. At first blush it appears to be clearly reserving these activities for physicians. On the other hand this subsection begins with the phrase "the related" which could mean the promotion of health, for example, must be related to the activity of assessing, diagnosing and treating individuals in order to constitute the practice of medicine. Finally, by including "other practices and procedures as taught at universities" it means activities that constitute the practice of medicine will vary with changes to medical school curricula. A particular problem is that nutrition is now taught as part of the curriculum of most medical schools including University of Toronto and Dalhousie. The need to know what is being taught

---

[16] Subsection 27(g) of the *Medical Act* contains an exemption for members of other Regulated Health Professions (such as Naturopaths) who practice within the scope of their authorized practice, provided they do not describe their activities as being the practice of medicine.

inside medical schools will make it very difficult or even impossible for the average person to know what constitutes the practice of medicine.

Until such time as a court interprets these provisions of the *Medical Act*, Holistic Nutritionists and other alternative therapy practitioners practicing in Nova Scotia face considerable uncertainty as to the scope of what they may lawfully do. Under Nova Scotia's *Summary Proceedings Act, R.S.* a breach of the *Medical Act* can result in a fine of up to $2,000 and/or 6 months imprisonment.

The *Naturopathic Doctors Act* makes it an offence to practice naturopathy unless authorized to do so under the Act. This Act also defines the practice of naturopathy to be "the assessment of diseases, disorders and dysfunctions and the naturopathic diagnosis and treatment of diseases, disorders and dysfunctions using naturopathic techniques to promote, maintain or restore health." As the diagnosis and treatment of diseases and disorders by any method is already restricted by the *Medical Act* (as these activities are seen to be within the scope of the practice of medicine) this restriction in the *Naturopathic Doctors Act* does not further limit the area of practice that is presently available to Holistic Nutritionists in Nova Scotia. Accordingly, I have not included provisions from the Act in the legislative summaries below.

The rules governing the practice of dietitians, the profession which is closest in nature to Holistic Nutritionists, is undergoing change. The *Professional Dietitians Act* is to be replaced by a new *Dietitians Act*. Interestingly, while the new Act received Royal Assent in 2009 it has not yet (as this is being written) been proclaimed into force. Despite enquiries to relevant stakeholders, including the Nova Scotia Dietetic Association, I have been unable to determine the reason for or the meaning of this lengthy delay. To assist Holistic Nutritionists with their planning material provisions from both the existing (and still in force) *Professional Dietitians Act* and the new (and not yet implemented) *Dietitians Act* are included in the legislative summaries below.

The *Professional Dietitians Act* does not define the practice of dietetics nor grant exclusive right to practice to registered dietitians. As a result, the current rules do not restrict the practice of a Holistic Nutritionist. The rules do, however, reserve several titles for exclusive use by registered dietitians, including "Dietitian" and "Nutritionist" and several variations. As the use of "Nutritionist" is prohibited, Holistic Nutritionists may not use it as part of a professional title in Nova Scotia. A breach of the *Professional Dietitians Act* can result in a fine of up to two thousand dollars, and in default of payment, to imprisonment for up to six months.

By contrast, the rules in the incoming *Dietitians Act* both expansively define the practice area of a registered dietitian <u>and</u> prohibit unregistered persons from providing such services to the public. For example, section 2 of the new Act defines the practice of dietetics to include: "planning, implementation and evaluation of nutrition interventions aimed at promoting health and preventing disease." Section 23 prohibits anyone from providing this service, unless registered under the new Act. The new rules also include the broad restrictions on professional titles contained in the old rules. A breach of the new *Dietitians Act,* once in force, will result in a fine of up to $2,000, and/or imprisonment for a term of up to 6 months. In addition, under subsection 31(5) of the new *Dietitians Act,* the onus will be on the accursed to prove he or she had the right to practice dietetics or that an exemption should apply.

As a result of the rules contained in the *Medical Act*, in particular its problematic definition of "practice of medicine", I believe there is considerable doubt as to whether a Holistic Nutritionist can lawfully carry on a conventional nutritional counselling practice in the province of Nova Scotia. This uncertain situation will become iron clad once the new *Dietitians Act* is proclaimed into force. One wishes the Nova Scotia legislature would have heeded the wisdom of Appeals Justice Osler as articulated in *Ontario Medical Act*, R.S.O. 1897, c. 176 when commenting about the scope of the practice of medicine: "Nevertheless, we cannot say that the profession, wide as have been its conquests and extended the scope of its practice, has taken all knowledge of the art of healing for its province . . . ".

For a better understanding of how terms such as "practice of medicine" are to be interpreted, the reader should review the discussion of terminology in the next chapter.

### Restrictions on Activities in Nova Scotia

Medical Act
c. 38 of the Acts of 2011

s. 2 In this Act, unless the context otherwise requires,

(af) "practice of medicine" means the practices and procedures usually performed by a medical practitioner and includes

(i)     the art and science of the assessment, diagnosis or treatment of an individual,

(ii)    the related promotion of health and prevention of illness, and

(iii)   such other practices and procedures as taught in universities or schools approved by the Council for licensing purposes under this Act and regulation

s. 22 (1)  Except as provided in this Act and the regulations, no person, other than a medical practitioner shall

(a) publicly or privately, for hire, gain or hope of reward, practice or offer to practice medicine;

(b) hold himself or herself out in any way to be entitled to practice medicine; or

(c) assume any title or description implying or designed to lead the public to believe that that person is entitled to practice medicine including the titles "physician", "surgeon", "medical practitioner", "medical specialist", "surgical specialist" and "doctor" or any derivation thereof.

25 (1)  A person who violates this Act or the regulations is guilty of an offence, and the Summary Proceedings Act applies in addition to any penalty otherwise provided for in this Act or the regulations.


Professional Dietitians Act
c. 361  of the revised statutes, 1989


No applicable practice restrictions.


The Dietitians Act
c. 2 of the Acts of 2009
*(to replace the Professional Dietitians Act*
*on a date to be determined)*

s. 2 In this Act,

(x) "practice of dietetics" means the translation and application of scientific knowledge of food and nutrition to human health through

(i) comprehensive nutritional assessment to determine nutritional status, nutrition-related diagnosis and nutritional requirements of individuals or populations related to health status and disease,

(ii) the planning, implementation and evaluation of nutrition interventions aimed at promoting health and preventing disease,

(iii) nutrition prescription, including enteral and parenteral nutrition and the prescription or ordering of drugs or other agents to optimize nutrition status,

(iv) ordering parameters required to monitor nutrition interventions and evaluate nutrition outcomes,

(v) the provision of nutrition education and counselling to clients, families, colleagues and health-care professionals,

(vi) development and evaluation of policies that affect food, food security and nutrition as it relates to health status,

(vii) integration of food and nutrition principles in the development and management of food service systems,

(viii) such delegated medical functions as are approved in accordance with the Medical Act, and

(ix) such other aspects of dietetics as may be prescribed in regulations approved by the Governor in Council, and

(x) research, education, consultation, management, administration, regulation, policy or system development relevant to subclauses (i) to (ix);

(ao) "scope of practice of the profession" means the roles, functions and accountabilities that dietitians are educated and authorized to perform;

s. 21 (1) No person shall engage in the practice of dietetics or describe the person's activities as "dietetics", "nutrition therapy" or "diet therapy" unless such person

(a) holds an active-practising licence with or without restrictions or conditions;

(b) is the holder of a temporary licence with or without restrictions or conditions;

(c) is the holder of a candidate licence with or without restrictions or conditions; or

(d) is otherwise authorized to engage in the practice of dietetics as set out in this Act or the regulations.

(2) No person shall

(a) take or use the designations "Dietitian", "Registered Dietitian", "Nutritionist", "Professional Nutritionist", "Professional Dietitian", "R.D.", "P.Dt", "R.D.N." or any derivation, translation or abbreviation thereof; or

(b) describe the person's activities as "Dietetics", "Nutrition Therapy" or "Diet Therapy",

in the Province, either alone or in combination with other words, letters or descriptions to imply that the person is entitled to practice as a dietitian unless the person

(c) holds an active-practising licence with or without restrictions or conditions;

(d) is the holder of a temporary licence with or without restrictions or conditions; or

(e) is otherwise authorized to use such designation and to engage in the practice of dietetics as set out in this Act or the regulations.

(3) No person shall engage in the practice of dietetics or take or use the designation "Dietetic Intern" or any derivation, translation or abbreviation thereof unless the person is engaged in a practicum approved by the Board and is authorized by the administrators of the practicum or otherwise authorized pursuant to the regulations to engage in the practice of dietetics.

(4) No person shall engage in the practice of dietetics or take or use the designation "Candidate Dietitian" or any derivation, translation or abbreviation thereof unless the person meets the criteria for the issuing of a candidate licence pursuant to this Act and the regulations and is authorized pursuant to the regulations to engage in the practice of

dietetics.

(5) In any advertisement or publication, including business cards, websites or signage, no person shall take or use the designation "Registered Dietitian", "Dietitian", "Professional Nutritionist", "Nutritionist", "Dietetic Intern", "Candidate Dietitian" or any derivation, translation or abbreviation thereof, or shall describe the person's activities as "dietetics", "nutrition therapy" or "diet therapy" unless the referenced activity falls within the definition of the "practice of dietetics".

s. 31 (1) Every person who

>    (a) knowingly furnishes false information in any application under this Act or in any statement required to be furnished under this Act or the regulations;
>
>    (b) engages in the practice of dietetics in the Province without complying with Section 29;
>
>    (c) engages in the practice of dietetics in violation of any condition or limitation contained in the person's licence; or
>
>    (d) otherwise contravenes this Act or the regulations,

is guilty of an offence and liable on summary conviction to a fine of not more than two thousand dollars or to imprisonment for a term of not more than six months, or to both.

## Restrictions on Professional Titles in Nova Scotia

Professional Dietitians Act
c. 361 of the revised statutes, 1989
(to be replaced by the Dietitians Act c. 2
of the Acts of 2009 on a date to be determined)

Designation of professional dietitian

s. 12 (1) Every person licenced pursuant to this Act may use the designation "Dietitian" or "Dietician", "Dietitian-Nutritionist", "Nutritionist", "Professional Dietitian" or "Professional Dietician", "Professional Dietitian-Nutritionist", "Professional Nutritionist", "Dietetiste", "Dietetiste-Nutritionniste", "Dietitiste Professionelle", "Dieteticienne", "Nutritionniste" or the initials "P. Dt." or "Dt. P."

(2) A person not licensed under this Act who is not qualified for membership in the Association may not use any of the following titles or designations: "Dietitian" or "Dietician", "Dietitian-Nutritionist", "Nutritionist", "Professional Dietitian" or "Professional Dietician", "Professional Dietitian-Nutritionist", "Professional Nutritionist", "Dietetiste", "Dietetiste- Nutritionniste", "Dietetiste Professionelle", "Dieteticienne", "Nutritionniste" or the initials "P.Dt." or "Dt.P." either alone or in combination with other

words, letters or descriptions.

(3) Any person who violates subsection (2) or in any way represents that that person is a professional dietitian or who by false and fraudulent declaration attempts to procure registration under this Act, is guilty of an offence and liable on summary conviction to a fine not exceeding two thousand dollars and in default of payment to imprisonment for a period not exceeding six months. R.S., c. 361, s. 12; 1990, c. 43, s. 7.

## Ontario

The provision of health services in Ontario is regulated using a Restricted Activities framework primarily through the *Regulated Health Professions Act*, its regulations and the associated individual acts that create the various self-governing Regulated Health Professions.

Section 27 of the *Regulated Health Professions Act* establishes the Restricted Activities (called Controlled Acts in Ontario) that may be performed only by members of designated Regulated Health Professions. A person who is not a member of a designated Regulated Health Profession may not perform any of these procedures, unless the situation falls within one of the limited exceptions provided for by the Act. In addition, section 30 of the Act further prohibits anyone from treating or advising a person "in circumstances in which it is reasonably foreseeable that serious bodily harm may result from the treatment or advice or from an omission from them." Interestingly, the *Regulated Health Professions Act* does not prohibit providing treatment per se. So Holistic Nutritionists in Ontario are permitted to treat diseases and disorders provided they do not perform a specific Controlled Act (e.g., selling or compounding a drug) when doing so, and their actions do not pose a serious foreseeable risk of bodily harm. A breach of the Controlled Acts provisions of the *Regulated Health Professions Act* can lead to a fine of up to $25,000 and/or imprisonment for up to one year, for a first offence.

The Ontario *Medicine Act* does not restrict the practice of medicine, which makes sense, as Ontario regulates the provision of health services using a Restricted Activities framework. However, the Act does include a general prohibition against a person who is not a member of the College of Physicians and Surgeons, holding himself/herself out to be a person who is qualified to practice as an osteopath, physician or surgeon or in a specialty of medicine.

While the Ontario *Dietetics Act* includes a short definition of the practice of dietetics, it does not restrict, in any way, who may engage in such a practice. The Act does, however, reserve the title "Dietitian" for exclusive use by registered dietitians. As the use of the word "Nutritionist" is not in any way restricted in Ontario, Holistic Nutritionists may use it as part of a professional title or in their marketing literature.

At the time this is being written, there is considerable debate within Ontario's complimentary health therapy industry about the pending implementation of a new Controlled Act dealing with the practice of psychotherapy techniques. This Controlled Act is defined to be:

> Treating, by means of psychotherapy technique, delivered through a therapeutic relationship, an individual's serious disorder of thought, cognition, mood, emotional regulation, perception or memory that may seriously impair the individual's judgement, insight, behaviour, communication or social functioning.[17]

The concern among critics is that the term "psychotherapy technique" is not defined and that a "therapeutic relationship" can be reasonably interpreted to include any client relationship that involves counselling or coaching services, such as many Holistic Nutritionists provide to their clients. The difficulty with this interpretation is that it ignores the conjunctive nature of this definition and looks selectively at only two of the four conditions it contains. For a treatment to be a Controlled Act under this section all four conditions must exist: (1) the use of a psychotherapy technique, *delivered* (2) within a therapeutic relationship, *to* (3) treat a serious disorder, etc., *that may* (4) seriously impair the individual's judgement, etc. Provided a Holistic Nutritionist is not treating a serious disorder that may seriously impair a client's judgement or behaviour, for example, he or she is free to use a technique with a client, such as counselling, even if it would constitute a "psychotherapy technique" being provided in a "therapeutic relationship."

A Holistic Nutritionist in Ontario who is not a member of a Regulated Health Profession may carry on a conventional nutritional counselling practice provided he or she: (1) does not perform any of the Controlled Acts described in the *Regulated Health Professions Act*; (2) does not provide advice or treatment where it is reasonably foreseeable serious bodily harm may result; (3) does not market themselves to the public using a title reserved for dietitians, or any another Regulated Health Profession; and (4) otherwise complies with laws of general application.

For a better understanding of how terms such as "diagnose" are to be interpreted, the reader should review the discussion of terminology in the next chapter.

---

[17] s. 27(2).14 *Regulated Health Professions Act*

## Restrictions on Activities in Ontario

Regulated Health Professions Act
1991 S.O. 1991, c. 18

Controlled acts restricted

s. 27. (1) No person shall perform a controlled act set out in subsection (2) in the course of providing health care services to an individual unless,

(a) the person is a member authorized by a health profession Act to perform the controlled act; or

(b) the performance of the controlled act has been delegated to the person by a member described in clause (a). 1991, c. 18, s. 27 (1); 1998, c. 18, Sched. G, s. 6.

Controlled acts

(2) A "controlled act" is any one of the following done with respect to an individual:

1. Communicating to the individual or his or her personal representative a diagnosis identifying a disease or disorder as the cause of symptoms of the individual in circumstances in which it is reasonably foreseeable that the individual or his or her personal representative will rely on the diagnosis.

2. Performing a procedure on tissue below the dermis, below the surface of a mucous membrane, in or below the surface of the cornea, or in or below the surfaces of the teeth, including the scaling of teeth.

3. Setting or casting a fracture of a bone or a dislocation of a joint.

4. Moving the joints of the spine beyond the individual's usual physiological range of motion using a fast, low amplitude thrust.

5. Administering a substance by injection or inhalation.

6. Putting an instrument, hand or finger,

    i. beyond the external ear canal,

    ii. beyond the point in the nasal passages where they normally narrow,

    iii. beyond the larynx,

    iv. beyond the opening of the urethra,

    v. beyond the labia majora,

    vi. beyond the anal verge, or

    vii. into an artificial opening into the body.

7. Applying or ordering the application of a form of energy prescribed by the regulations under this Act.

8. Prescribing, dispensing, selling or compounding a drug as defined in the *Drug and Pharmacies Regulation Act*[18], or supervising the part of a pharmacy where such

drugs are kept.

9. Prescribing or dispensing, for vision or eye problems, subnormal vision devices, contact lenses or eye glasses other than simple magnifiers.

10. Prescribing a hearing aid for a hearing impaired person.

11. Fitting or dispensing a dental prosthesis, orthodontic or periodontal appliance or a device used inside the mouth to protect teeth from abnormal functioning.

12. Managing labour or conducting the delivery of a baby.

13. Allergy challenge testing of a kind in which a positive result of the test is a significant allergic response. 1991, c. 18, s. 27 (2); 2007, c. 10, Sched. L, s. 32.

Note: On a day to be named by proclamation of the Lieutenant Governor, subsection (2) is amended by the Statutes of Ontario, 2007, chapter 10, Schedule R, subsection 19 (1) by adding the following paragraph:

14. Treating, by means of psychotherapy technique, delivered through a therapeutic relationship, an individual's serious disorder of thought, cognition, mood, emotional regulation, perception or memory that may seriously impair the individual's judgement, insight, behaviour, communication or social functioning.

s. 29.1 (1) No person shall, in the course of providing health care services, provide any treatment that seeks to change the sexual orientation or gender identity of a person under 18 years of age. 2015, c. 18, s. 2.

s. 30. (1) No person, other than a member treating or advising within the scope of practice of his or her profession, shall treat or advise a person with respect to his or her health in circumstances in which it is reasonably foreseeable that serious bodily harm may result from the treatment or advice or from an omission from them. 1991, c. 18, s. 30 (1); 2007, c. 10, Sched. M, s. 6.

40. (1) Every person who contravenes subsection 27 (1), 29.1 (1) or 30 (1) is guilty of an offence and on conviction is liable,

(a) for a first offence, to a fine of not more than $25,000, or to imprisonment for a term of not more than one year, or both; and

(b) for a second or subsequent offence, to a fine of not more than $50,000, or to imprisonment for a term of not more than one year, or both. 2007, c. 10, Sched. M, s. 12; 2015, c. 18, s. 3.

Medicine Act
1991 S.O. 1991, c. 30

---

[18] Natural health products, as defined in the *Natural Health Products Regulations* to Canada's *Food and Drug Act* are not considered drugs under the *Drug and Pharmacies Regulation Act*.

s. 9 (3) No person other than a member shall hold himself or herself out as a person who is qualified to practice in Ontario as an osteopath, physician or surgeon or in a specialty of medicine. 1991, c. 30, s. 9 (3).

## Restrictions on Professional Titles in Ontario

Dietetics Act
1991 S.O. 1991, c. 26

s. 3 The practice of dietetics is the assessment of nutrition and nutritional conditions and the treatment and prevention of nutrition related disorders by nutritional means.

s. 7 (1) No person other than a member shall use the title "dietitian", a variation or abbreviation or an equivalent in another language. 1991, c. 26, s. 7 (1).

(2) No person other than a member shall hold himself or herself out as a person who is qualified to practice in Ontario as a dietitian or in a specialty of dietetics. 1991, c. 26, s. 7 (2).

## Prince Edward Island

The provision of health services in Prince Edward Island is regulated using a Professional Exclusivity framework. The rules that impact the practices of Holistic Nutritionists are primarily drawn from the *Medical Act* and the *Dietitians Act*. Naturopathy is not a Regulated Health Profession in P.E.I.

Section 56 of the *Medical Act* makes it an offence to practice or to hold yourself out as being qualified to practice medicine unless licensed to do so under the Act. Section 1 of the *Medical Act* contains an illustrative list of practice areas (e.g., surgery, obstetrics) that are deemed to be included within the meaning of "medicine." As the definition of the practice of medicine in the Act does not include any defined activities, the question of whether in providing services a Holistic Nutritionist is practising medicine would be determined by the courts, although practising medicine is generally interpreted to include, among other things, diagnosing and treating diseases and disorders. A breach of the *Medical Act* can result in a fine of up to $5,000, and/or imprisonment for a term of up to six months.

The *Dietitians Act* defines the scope of a registered dietitian's practice. While it does not restrict an unregulated professional from carrying on a dietitian's practice, it does makes it unlawful for unregulated professionals to hold themselves out as being registered dietitians who are entitled to engage in the practice of dietetics. The *Dietitians Act* reserves the title "Dietitian" and several related variations for exclusive use by registered dietitians. It also prohibits anyone who is not a registered dietitian from using any title, etc. that implies he or she is a registered dietitian. As the Act does not restrict in any way the use of the title "Nutritionist," Holistic Nutritionists may use it as part of a professional title and in their advertising and marketing literature. A breach of these provisions in the *Dietitians Act* can result in a fine of up to $2,000.

A Holistic Nutritionist who is not a member of a Regulated Health Profession in P.E.I may carry on a conventional nutritional counselling practice provided he or she: (1) does not practice medicine as this term is defined in the *Medical Act* and has been interpreted by the courts; (2) does not market themselves to the public using a title reserved for registered dietitians or any another Regulated Health Profession or otherwise falsely represent themselves as being a registered dietitian or member of another Regulated Health Profession; and (3) otherwise complies with laws of general application.

For a better understanding of how the courts have interpreted "practice of medicine" as well as other relevant terms, the reader should review the discussion of terminology in the next chapter.

## Restrictions on Activities in Prince Edward Island

Medical Act
SNL 2005 c. M-4.01

s. 1 In this Act

(q) "practice of medicine" means the practice of medicine, surgery, obstetrics, pathology, radiology and the specialities thereof, but does not include veterinary surgery

s. 56 (1) Except as provided in this Act, and the regulations, no person, other than a medical practitioner who holds a license or a professional corporation which holds a license, shall

(a) publicly or privately, for hire, gain or hope of reward, practice or offer to practice medicine;

(b) hold himself or itself out in any way to be entitled to practice medicine; or

(c) assume any title or description implying or designed to lead the public to believe that he or it is entitled to practice medicine.

(2) No person is entitled to receive a fee, reward or remuneration for professional services rendered or medicine or medical supplies supplied to any person in the practice of Medicine unless registered and licensed at the time the services were provided, or medicine or supplies were.

s. 62. A person who violates an order made under section 32.8, sections 55 to 60 or any provision of a regulation the contravention of which constitutes an offence is liable on summary conviction to a fine not exceeding $5,000, or to imprisonment for a term not exceeding six months, or both. 1987,c.47,s.62; 1997,c.30,s.16 {eff.} Sept. 8/98.

## Restrictions on Professional Titles in Prince Edward Island

Dietitians Act
c. D-10.1

s. 1 In this Act

(e) "dietetics" means the professional practice of applying scientific knowledge of foods and nutrition to human health and, in particular,

(i) assessing the nutritional status and requirements of individuals or groups of individuals,

(ii) designing general standards and determining care plans appropriate to meet nutritional requirements,

(iii) designing, evaluating and communicating to the public, information on nutrition matters for the purposes of health education and consumer protection,

(iv) directing nutritional therapy,

(v) ensuring the nutritional quality and safety of food service in a health-care institution or program;

(f) "dietitian" means a person registered under this Act

s. 20 No person other than a registered dietitian holding a valid certificate shall

(a) engage in or carry on the practice of dietetics under the title of "dietitian", "RD", "P.Dt.", "dietetiste", "Dt.p" or such other similar designation as may be prescribed in regulations;

(b) call herself or himself a "registered dietitian", "RD", "P.Dt.", "dietetiste professionelle", "Dt.p." or other similar designation as may be prescribed; or

(c) take or use any name, title, or description implying or calculated to lead people to infer that the person is a registered dietitian.

s. 21. Anyone who violates section 20 is guilty of an offence and is liable on summary conviction to a fine not exceeding $2,000.

# Quebec

The provision of health services in Quebec is regulated using a Restricted Activities framework. The rules that impact the practices of Holistic Nutritionists are primarily drawn from the *Medical Act* and the *Professional Code* which defines the profession of dietetics in Quebec and establishes the "Ordre professionnel des diététistes du Québec" as the regulatory body for dietitians. Naturopathy is not a Regulated Health Profession in Quebec.

The *Medical Act* defines the practice of medicine and establishes a list of reserved activities (i.e., Restricted Activities) that may only be performed by members of the medical profession duly licensed under the Act. In reviewing the reserved activities, the reader will see that diagnosing illness, determining medical treatment, prescribing medications and other substances, and prescribing treatment are all reserved. In understanding the meaning of "determining medical treatment," reference must also be made back to the broad definition of the practice of medicine included in the *Medical Act:* "The practice of medicine consists in assessing and diagnosing any deficiency in health and in preventing and treating illness to maintain or restore the health of a person in interaction with his environment."

The unlawful performance of a reserved activity under the *Medical Act* by an individual can result in a fine of up to $20,000 for a first offence.

The *Professional Code* defines the practice of dietetics and section 37 identifies two procedures that may only be performed by members of the Ordre professionnel des diététistes du Québec. These procedures involve determining a nutritional plan where "an individual prescription indicates that nutrition is a determining factor in the treatment of illness" and monitoring the nutritional status of a person who is on such a plan. The use of the word "prescription," which the *Medical Act* defines to be within the exclusive purview of a physician (see the *Medical Act* s 35(6) below) indicates the nutritional plan must be prescribed by a physician as part of the treatment of a disease to become a reserved act (i.e., Restricted Activity) of members of the Ordre professionnel des diététistes du Quebec.

Section 36 of the *Professional Code* also reserves several titles for exclusive use by members of the Ordre professionnel des dietetistes du Québec, including "Dietitian" and "Nutritionist," several related abbreviations, and any other title that may wrongfully imply a person is a member of the Order.

A breach of a provision of the Professional Code by an individual can result in a fine of up to $20,000 for a first offence.

A Holistic Nutritionist who is not a member of a Regulated Health Profession in Quebec may carry on a conventional nutritional counselling practice provided he or she: (1) does not perform any reserved activities (i.e., Restricted Activities) which includes diagnosing and treating diseases and disorders; (2) does not market themselves to the public using "Dieician", "Dietitian" or "Nutritionist" or another a title reserved for members of the Ordre professionnel des diététistes du Québec or any another Regulated Health Profession; and (3) otherwise complies with laws of general application.

Quebec establishes reserved activities on a profession by profession basis. I have summarized activities that are reserved for physicians and dietitians. The *Professional Code* provisions for other Regulated Health Professions should be consulted if your practice includes activities other than providing general nutritional counselling to promote health and wellness, or if you provide any other services that you suspect may be an activity commonly practiced by another Regulated Health Profession in Quebec.

For a better understanding of how terms such as "diagnose" and "treat" are to be interpreted, the reader should review the discussion of terminology in the following chapter.

### Restrictions on Activities in Quebec

Medical Act
R.S.Q., chapter M-9

s. 31. The practice of medicine consists in assessing and diagnosing any deficiency in health and in preventing and treating illness to maintain or restore the health of a person in interaction with his environment.

Reserved activities.

The following activities in the practice of medicine are reserved to physicians:

> (1) diagnosing illnesses;
>
> (2) prescribing diagnostic examinations;
>
> (3) using diagnostic techniques that are invasive or entail risks of injury;
>
> (4) determining medical treatment;
>
> (5) prescribing medications and other substances;
>
> (6) prescribing treatment;
>
> (7) using techniques or applying treatments that are invasive or entail risks of injury, including aesthetic procedures;
>
> (8) providing clinical monitoring of the condition of patients whose state of health is problematic;

(9) providing pregnancy care and conducting deliveries;

(10) making decisions as to the use of restraint measures; and

(11) deciding to use isolation measures in accordance with the Act respecting health services and social services (chapter S-4.2) and the Act respecting health services and social services for Cree Native persons (chapter S-5).

s. 43. Subject to the rights and privileges expressly granted by law to other professionals, no person may engage in any activity described in the second paragraph of section 31, unless he is a physician.

s. 45. Every person who contravenes any provision of section 43 is liable, for each offence, to the penalties provided in section 188 of the Professional Code (chapter C-26).

Professional Code
C-26,

s. 37 Every member of one of the following professional orders may engage in the following professional acidities in addition to those otherwise allowed him by law:

(c) the Ordre professionnel des dietetistes du Quebec: assess the nutritional status of a person and determine and ensure the implementation of a response strategy designed to tailor diet to needs in order to maintain or restore health.

s. 37.1 Every member of one of the following professional orders may engage in the following professional activities, which are reserved to such members with the scope of the activities they may engage under section 37

(1) the Ordre professionnel des diététistes du Québec:

  (a) determine a nutritional plan, including the appropriate feeding route, where an individual prescription indicates that nutrition is a determining factor in the treatment of illness; and

  (b) monitor the nutritional status of persons whose nutritional treatment plan has been determined

s. 37.2 A person shall not in any manner engage in a professional activity reserved under section s. 37.1 to members of a professional order, claim to have the right to do so or act in such a way as to lead to the belief that the person is authorized to do so, unless the person holds a valid, appropriate permit and is entered on the roll of the order empowered to issue the permit except if it is allowed by law.

s. 38 Nothing in this division shall be interpreted as giving to members of an order to which it applies the exclusive right to engage in the activities described in section 37, in letters patent constituting such order or in an amalgamation or integration order.

s. 188. Every person who contravenes a provision of this Code, of the Act or letters patent constituting an order or of an amalgamation or integration order is guilty of an offence and is liable to a fine of not less than $1,500 nor more than $20,000 or, in the case of a legal person, of not less than $3,000 nor more than $40,000.

In the case of a subsequent offence, the minimum and maximum fines are doubled.

## Restrictions on Professional Titles in Quebec

Professional Code
C-26,

s. 36 No person shall in any way whatsoever;

(c) use the title "Dieician", "Dietitian" or "Nutritionist" or any other title or abbreviation which may lead to the belief that his is a dietician, a dietitian or a nutritionist, or use initials which may lead to the belief that he is a dietician, dietitian or a nutritionist, or the initials "P.Dt.", "Dt.P" or "R.D." unless he holds a valid permit for that purpose and is entered on the roll of the Ordre professionnel des dietetistes du Quebec.

# Saskatchewan

The rules that impact the practices of Holistic Nutritionists in Saskatchewan are primarily drawn from the *Medical Profession Act*, the *Naturopathic Act* and the *Dietitians Act*.

Section 5 of the *Medical Profession Act* makes it an offence for anyone who is not a member of the College of Physicians and Surgeons of Saskatchewan to, among other things, engage in or profess to engage in any aspect of the practice of medicine, or to furnish any medicine or treat any disease or ailment by medicine for hire, gain or hope of reward. As "practice of medicine" is not defined by the statute, the question of whether in providing services a Holistic Nutritionist is practising medicine would be determined by the courts, but it would certainly include the activities of treating diseases and disorders, furnishing medicines, etc. as specified by the Act. A breach of the *Medical Profession Act* can result in a fine of up to $5,000 for a first offence.

The *Naturopathic Act* makes it an offence to practice naturopathy or use the title "Naturopath," etc. unless authorized to do so under the Act. This Act also defines the practice of naturopathy to be "the art of healing by natural methods as taught in recognized schools of naturopathy." While the "art of healing" is not defined in the statute, common sense implies it should mean, at a minimum, diagnosing and treating diseases and disorders. The reference to "healing by natural methods as taught in recognized schools of naturopathy" is more problematic. Healing by natural means could include diet, exercise, and by use of Natural Health Products. But whether it does is a function of whether their use as healing practices are taught in recognized schools of naturopathy. The need to know what is being taught inside schools makes it very difficult or even impossible for Holistic Nutritionists to know what constitutes the practice of naturopathy in Saskatchewan.

It may be of some comfort to Holistic Nutritionists to know that the Supreme Court of Canada has determined that statutes that create professional monopolies are to be strictly construed "so that anything which is not clearly prohibited to non-members of the profession may be done by them."[19] It could be argued that this interpretive guideline tips the scales in favour of Holistic Nutritionists. A breach of the *Naturopathic Act* can result in a fine of up to $100 for a first offence.

As this is being written, Saskatchewan is in the process of updating the *Naturopathic Act*. If Bill 178 passes and comes into force the problems associated with the current definition of naturopathy will no longer exist as the Bill does not link the definition to what is being taught in schools. I have set out key sections from the proposed Bill at the end of this section.

---

[19] R. v. Windrum. See also Laporte v. Collège des Pharmaciens (Québec) (1974), 23 C.C.C. (2d) 45.

The *Dietitians Act* does not define the practice of dietetics nor restrict in any way who may carry on a nutritional consulting practice. The Act reserves the title "Dietitian" and several related variations for exclusive use by registered dietitians. It also prohibits anyone who is not a registered dietitian from using any title, etc. that implies he or she is a registered dietitian. As the Act does not restrict in any way the use of the title "Nutritionist," Holistic Nutritionists may use it as part of a professional title and in their marketing and advertising. A breach of the *Dietitians Act* can result in a fine of up to $2,000 for a first offence.

As noted above, an argument can be made that the practice of a Holistic Nutritionist in Saskatchewan falls within the exclusive practice scope of registered naturopaths. Unfortunately, I was unable to locate any reported court decisions directly reviewing this question. Subject to this qualification, a Holistic Nutritionist who is not a member of a Regulated Health Profession in Saskatchewan may carry on a conventional nutritional practice provided he or she: (1) does not practice medicine as this term is defined in the *Medical Act* and has been interpreted by the courts, or otherwise furnish medicine or treat any disease, etc. by medicine for a fee; (2) does not practice naturopathy as this term is defined in the *Naturopathic Act*; (3) does not market themselves to the public using a title reserved for registered dietitians, or another Regulated Health Profession or otherwise falsely represent themselves as being a registered dietitian, or member of another Regulated Health Profession, and (4) otherwise complies with laws of general application.

For a better understanding of how terms such as "practice of medicine," etc. are to be interpreted, the reader should review the discussion of terminology in next chapter.

### Restrictions on Activities in Saskatchewan

The Medical Profession Act
1981c. M-10.1 of the Statutes of Saskatchewan, 1980-81

Interpretation

s. 2 In this Act

(k) "practice" means the practice of medicine, surgery or midwifery

s. 80(1) A person who is not registered under this Act and who:

>      (a) for hire, gain or hope of reward:

>>           (i) engages in, professes to engage in or advertises to give advice in any aspect of practice; or

>>           (ii) furnishes any medicine or treats any disease or ailment by medicine, drugs or any Form of treatment, influence or appliance;

(b) takes or uses any name, title, addition or description representing, implying or calculated to lead people to infer that he is registered under this Act to practice, or that he is recognized by law as a physician, surgeon or podiatric surgeon;

(c) assumes, uses or employs the term "doctor", "surgeon", "physician" or "podiatric surgeon" or any affix or prefix indicative of any such title as an occupational designation that relates to the treatment of human ailments, or advertises or holds himself out as such;

(d) pretends to be a physician, doctor of medicine, surgeon, podiatric surgeon, practitioner or healer of the sick; or

(e) assumes any title, addition or description other than that which he actually possesses and is legally entitled to use under this Act;

is guilty of an offence and liable on summary conviction, in the case of a first offence, to a fine of not more than $5,000, in the case of a second offence, to a fine of not more than $10,000, and, in the case of a third or subsequent offence, to a fine of not more than $15,000.


The Naturopathy Act

Being Chapter N-4 of The Revised Statutes of Saskatchewan, 1978 (effective February 26, 1979) as amended by the Statutes of Saskatchewan, 1980-81, c.21 and 62; 1984-85-86, c.16; 1989-90, c.54 and 1994, c.P-37.1; 2004, c.L-16.1; and 2010, c.B-12 and c.19.

s. 2 In this Act:

(d) "naturopathic practitioner" means a person who is registered as such under this Act;

(e) "naturopathy" means the art of healing by natural methods as taught in recognized schools of naturopathy.

s. 9 No person, other than a naturopathic practitioner registered under this Act as a member of the association shall engage in the practice of naturopathy or use the title "Naturopathic Practitioner", "Naturopath", "Doctor of Naturopathy" or any word, title or designation, abbreviated or otherwise, to imply that he is engaged in the practice of naturopathy, and every person who contravenes this section is guilty of an offence against this Ac Prohibition against unauthorized practice

s. 11(1) Every person who practices naturopathy, either alone or in conjunction with any other method of treatment of the human body for disease and the causes of disease, for hire, gain, reward or remuneration, or the hope or expectation thereof, unless he is duly registered to practice as a naturopath under this Act is guilty of an offence against this Act.

(2) Every person who, not being registered as a naturopathic practitioner under this Act, or who, having been so registered and whose registration has been cancelled or is under suspension, practices or holds himself out as practising naturopathy, either alone or in conjunction with any other method of treatment of the human body for disease and the causes of disease, or advertises or uses any prefix or suffix to his name signifying that he is qualified to practice naturopathy either alone or in conjunction with any other method of treatment of

the human body for disease and the causes of disease, is guilty of an offence against this Act.

s. 12 Every person who is guilty of an offence against this Act is, on summary conviction, liable for a first offence to a fine not exceeding $100, for a second offence to a fine not exceeding $250, and for a subsequent offence to imprisonment for a period not exceeding three months, without the option of a fine.

BILL No. 172
An Act respecting the Practice of Naturopathic Medicine
and the College of Naturopathic Doctors of Saskatchewan

s. 24(1) Subject to the terms and conditions of a member's licence, a member may perform the following authorized practices:

(a) assessing, monitoring and treating an individual's symptoms, disease, disorder or condition using the techniques, therapies and therapeutics of naturopathic medicine;

(b) communicating a naturopathic medical diagnosis identifying, as the cause of an individual's symptoms, a disease, disorder or condition that may be identified through an assessment using the techniques, therapies and therapeutics of naturopathic medicine;

(c) for the purposes of clauses (a) and (b):

(i) prescribing or administering drugs in accordance with the regulatory bylaws and the regulations made pursuant to The Pharmacy Act, 1996;

(ii) ordering, performing, accessing, interpreting or using medical laboratory tests in accordance with the regulatory bylaws made pursuant to this Act and the regulations made pursuant to The Medical Laboratory Licensing Act, 1994;

(iii) performing invasive procedures that are prescribed in the bylaws.

(2) No person shall engage in the business or practice of performing any of the authorized practices described in subsection (1) with respect to another individual unless:

(a) the person is a member who is authorized by his or her licence to perform that practice;

(b) the person is authorized pursuant to another Act to perform that practice;

(c) the person is administering first aid or temporary assistance in cases of emergency; or

(d) the person is treating human ailments by prayer or spiritual means as an enjoyment or exercise of religious freedom.

s. 45 Every person who contravenes section 22 or 24 is guilty of an offence and liable on summary conviction:

(a) for a first offence, to a fine of not more than $5,000;

(b) for a second offence, to a fine of not more than $10,000; and

(c) for each subsequent offence, to a fine of not more than $15,000.

## Restrictions on Professional Titles in Saskatchewan

The Dietitians Act
c. D-27.1 of the Statutes of Saskatchewan, 2001

Protection of title

s. 21 No person other than a member shall use the title "Dietitian", "Registered Dietitian" or "Professional Dietitian" or the abbreviation "R.D." or "P.Dt." or any word, title or designation, abbreviated or otherwise, to imply that the person is a member.

Offence and penalty

s. 40 Every person who contravenes section 21 is guilty of an offence and liable on summary conviction:

(a) for a first offence, to a fine of not more than $2,000;

(b) for a second offence, to a fine of not more than $4,000; and

(c) for each subsequent offence, to a fine of not more than $6,000, to imprisonment for a term of not more than six months or to both.

# Chapter 4
# Interpreting Key Terms

In the previous chapter I reviewed the rules that most directly restrict the right of a Holistic Nutritionist to carry on a conventional nutritional consulting practice in the various Canadian provinces. To more fully understand the scope of the law, however, it is also necessary to look at the meanings of the key words and phrases used in these rules. For example, while it is useful to know that Holistic Nutritionists in the provinces of Manitoba[20], New Brunswick, Newfoundland and Labrador, Nova Scotia[21], Prince Edward Island and Saskatchewan can generally provide nutritional counselling services provided they do not engage in the "practice of medicine," this information is far more useful if we also understand what activities are included within "the practice of medicine." The same goes for other key terms used throughout the laws of the different provinces: "diagnosis," "diseases and disorders," "drug," and "treatment."

Sometimes words and phrases are defined within the statute relying on their use. When this is the case, the statute can be understood with the highest degree of certainty. For example, the Nova Scotia *Medical Act* defines the practice of medicine to include "the art and science of the assessment, diagnosis or treatment of an individual." So in this province, we know with absolute certainty that the "practice of medicine" includes these activities.

When a statute does not provide this guidance we must search to see how the words and phrases have been interpreted by judges over the years, in legal dictionaries, and in legislation of other provinces. The answers provided by this research can be a good indicator of how a court may proceed but cannot be determinative. Courts can and do interpret the same words and phrases in

---

[20] Manitoba is currently in the process of changing how it regulates Health Professions. An overview of the changes it is implementing can be found in Chapter 3.

[21] The Nova Scotia *Medical Act* contains a somewhat unique definition practice of medicine and must be carefully reviewed if you provide complementary health therapy services in this province.

different ways, sometimes even reaching quite conflicting decisions. This can happen for many reasons, including the personalities of the judges involved and the different facts that exist in the cases before them. In one set of facts, their sense of justice may direct them towards interpreting a word or phrase broadly, in another, narrowly. As troublesome as this uncertainty is for Holistic Nutritionists, it is a fact of life.

This point was well illustrated in the Sandhar case, which I first mentioned in Chapter 2. The reader may recall this case involved a homeopath in Alberta who prescribed a liver cleanser as treatment for an inflamed liver, which he diagnosed using a machine that measured the flow of energy of various organs from acqua pressure meridian points. I believe it is safe to say this was not a diagnostic procedure, diagnosis or treatment likely to have been followed by a conventional physician operating in Alberta at that time. Perhaps it is for this reason that the trial judge found Mr. Sandhar not guilty of practising medicine. The judges on appeal, however, took a different view and found Mr. Sandhar guilty.

The facts of a case have a very important impact on the result. In the words of former Chief Justice Moss, of the Ontario Court of Appeal[22] while considering whether the phrase "practice of medicine" means an attempt to cure or alleviate disease by the use of drugs:

> But unless there is a concrete case with the facts proved or known, how is it possible to say whether or not the words of sec. 49 are applicable? If the answer given was that if it were shewn [sic] that a person not registered under the Ontario *Medical Act* attempted to cure or alleviate disease by methods and course of treatment known to medical science and adopted and used in their practice by medical practitioners registered under the Act, or advised or prescribed treatment for disease or illness such as would be advised or prescribed by the registered practitioner, then, although what was done, prescribed or administered did not involve the use or application of any drug or other substance having or supposed to have the property of curing or alleviating disease, he might be held to be practising medicine with the meaning of section 49, it would still leave the matter to be dealt with in a concrete case, in which the ultimate decision must turn upon the facts found.

So with this bit of guidance in mind, let's see how some key words and phrases have been defined by the courts and in the legal literature to gain a better idea of how they may be interpreted and applied in the future.

---

[22] Ontario Medical Act, Re (1906) 13 O.L.R. 501 (Ed. this Act has now been rescinded)

## Diagnosis

Within all Canadian provinces, with the exception of Alberta, the right to lawfully make a diagnosis is restricted to one or more Regulated Health Professions. It very important to understand, therefore, what making a diagnosis means. Here are some of the ways this term has been defined:

> The identification of a disease by means of a patient's symptoms.[23]

> To determine the nature of the disease or disorder in a given case.[24]

> The determination of what kind of disease a patient is suffering from, especially the art of distinguishing between several possibilities. Also, the verdict (the name of the disease) decided upon.[25]

The Sandhar decision, referred to previously, also provides instruction about what it means to make a diagnosis. In this case, a homeopath was found to have made a diagnosis even though he used an energy test to identify liver and lung inflammation resulting from a buildup of toxins. This decision illustrates the point that someone can be found to have provided a diagnosis even if they used diagnostic procedures that are outside the normal practice of conventional medicine. What matters is not the procedures used, but rather the results achieved—the determination or identification of a disease or disorder the patient is suffering from. Here is a quote from the decision:

> The Respondent [ed. Sandhar] examined Miss Lewis and stated to her that she had lung congestion and liver and kidney inflammation. That act, on his part, fits directly within s. 77(1) (a) in that he stated an ability or willingness to diagnose a human disease or illness. Dr. LeRiche gave evidence that these two complaints were in fact illness.

The term "diagnosis" is very broadly defined and is not connected to any particular process or health modality. Instead, it hinges on the rendering of a conclusion or verdict that an individual is suffering from a disease, or disorder.

## Diseases & Disorders

Legislation that regulates the act of making a diagnosis links it to making a diagnosis of a disease or disorder. Once again, you will see these terms are broadly defined and can logically be

---

[23] R. v. Windrum
[24] J. E. Schmidt, *Attorney's Dictionary of Medicine* (New York: Mathew Bender and Company, Inc., 2005)
[25] Ibid.

interpreted to include virtually any deviation from what is considered to be the healthy norm, including resulting from nutritional deficiencies.

> Disease – An unhealthy condition of the body (or a part of it) or the mind; illness, sickness[26]

> Disease – 1. Morbus; illness; sickness; an interruption, cessation or disorder of bodily functions, systems, or organs. 2. A morbid entity characterized by at least two of these criteria, recognized etiologic agent(s) identifiable group of signs and symptoms or consistent anatomical alterations.[27]

> Disorder – A condition marked by deviation from normal activity or function; a disease; an abnormal mental or physical condition.[28]

> Disorder – A disturbance of function, structure or both resulting from a genetic or embryonic failure in development or from exogenous factors such as poison, trauma or disease.[29]

## Drug

Directly or indirectly, the action of prescribing a drug is restricted to physicians and members of certain other Regulated Health Professions in all provinces. Understanding what is and is not considered a drug in the province in which you practice is relevant for all Holistic Nutritionists.

Restricted Activity Framework

Within provinces that regulate using a Restricted Activities framework, the prescribing or dispensing of drugs[30] is universally a Restricted Activity. While the rules vary somewhat from province to province, a drug, for purposes of Restricted Activities, is generally defined to mean a substance that is either illegal, requires a prescription, or otherwise controlled—meaning that it must be sold under the supervision of a pharmacist[31]. If you think about it, this threshold makes sense. The purpose in regulating using a Restricted Activity framework is to only restrict activities that are deemed risky. If a substance is freely available over the counter for purchase

---

[26] R. v. Windrum.

[27] William R. Hensyl, ed., *Stedman's Medical Dictionary*, 25th ed. (Baltimore: Williams & Wilkins, 1990).

[28] J. E. Schmidt, *Attorney's Dictionary of Medicine* (New York: Mathew Bender and Company, Inc., 2005).

[29] William R. Hensyl, ed., *Stedman's Medical Dictionary*, 25th ed. (Baltimore: Williams & Wilkins, 1990).

[30] Quebec's *Medical Act,* R.S.Q. c. M-9 does not use the term "drug" and instead restricts "prescribing medications and substances" which are not defined in this Act. The discussion of the meaning of "Drug" in this section, therefore, does not apply to the rules in Quebec.

[31] General information on a drug's registration category can be found at the National Association of Pharmacy Regulatory Authorities website: http://napra.ca/pages/home/default.aspx (accessed June 4, 2015).

by consumers without the supervision of a physician or pharmacist, it must be of a type that carries minimal risk of harm even if used incorrectly. Accordingly, nothing is gained by prohibiting unlicensed and complimentary therapy practitioners from recommending them to their clients.

Holistic Nutritionists practicing in a province that regulates using the Restricted Activities framework may generally recommend over the counter medicines such as acetaminophen, Natural Health Products, and herbs and plants with healing properties (assuming they are otherwise lawfully available) to their clients without crossing the threshold of illegally prescribing drugs[32]. However, as there are some differences between how Restricted Activities provinces define a drug, (Ontario has slightly more stringent rules than Alberta, for example) the rules applicable in the province in which you practice must always be carefully reviewed.

Professional Exclusivity Framework

In provinces that regulate using a Professional Exclusivity framework prescribing a drug is restricted by virtue of being an aspect of the practice of medicine. In certain provinces the definition of practice of medicine provides for this directly. In other provinces it is part of the definition as a result of court decisions. In all cases, however, Holistic Nutritionists practicing in these provinces face the problem that neither the rules, nor the courts provide a definitive definition of what constitutes a drug for the purpose of being found to practice medicine. Common sense might tell us it includes prescription medications, as is the case in provinces that regulate using a Restricted Activities framework and that Holistic Nutritionists should avoid recommending such drugs (in any event doing so would be somewhat antithetical to the world view of most Holistic Nutritionists). But what about non-prescription substances? What about over the counter medications such as acetaminophen? What about Natural health Products? What about herbs and plants with healing properties? Do these substances constitute drugs for the purpose of being fund to practice medicine?

In one sense astute readers may feel this determination is a moot point. After all, in provinces that regulate through restricting the practice of medicine Holistic Nutritionists must also avoid treating diseases and disorders as this activity is also an aspect of the practice of medicine and one usually prescribes a substance for the purpose of providing a treatment. However, while this is usually true, it is not always true. In most provinces, Holistic Nutritionists may work with clients to improve their overall health and well-being, even if they are prohibited from recommending treatments for diseases and disorders. In doing so it may be useful to recommend

---

[32] Practitioners who reside in B.C. and Manitoba, however, still must concern themselves with whether in prescribing an otherwise legal substance, they are engaging in the Restricted Activity of recommending or providing a treatment of a disease or disorder.

substances that aid in improving health and vitality. So the question of knowing when a substance is a drug, remains relevant.

As Canadians, a logical starting place to start looking for a definition of "drug" is the federal *Food and Drugs Act*[33] which applies to the manufacturing, promotion and sale of all food and drugs in Canada.

The *Food and Drugs Act* defines a drug to include:

> any substance or mixture of substances manufactured, sold or represented for use in:

> (a) the diagnosis, treatment, mitigation or prevention of a disease, disorder or abnormal physical state, or its symptoms, in human beings or animals,

> (b) restoring, correcting or modifying organic functions in human beings or animals, or

> (c) disinfection in premises in which food is manufactured, prepared or kept;

By contrast it defines food to include:

> any article manufactured, sold or represented for use as food or drink for human beings, chewing gum, and any ingredient that may be mixed with food for any purpose whatever;

The frustrating thing about this Act is that all products that are consumed must be classified under these one of these two categories—and the determination of which category a substance falls into depends not upon what the substance is (e.g., a man-made chemical or agent) but rather what is said or represented about it. This strange reality was confirmed in Wrigley Canada v. R[34] where the Federal Court of Appeal determined that under the *Food and Drugs Act* a substance may be classified as both food and a drug at the same time, depending upon the representations made about it. As a result, chewing gum, which is expressly identified in the *Food and Drugs Act* to be food, was also seen to be a drug when the manufacturer sought to advertise that its "Extra" sugarless gum prevents tooth decay.

For Holistic Nutritionists trying to understand what they can and cannot recommend without crossing the threshold of practicing medicine, this obviously creates a problem. In any province where a drug is not otherwise defined, it is very logical to assume the definition contained in the federal *Food and Drugs Act* should apply and this definition clearly states that any substance, even one that is normally viewed to be food, becomes a drug when preventive or curative claims are made about it. Does this mean a Holistic Nutritionist who makes such a claim about food, or

---

[33] *Food and Drugs Act*, R.S., 1985, c. F-27
[34] Wrigley Canada v. R. (2000) 96 A.C.W.S. (3d) 888

who recommends a product that has such a claim contained on its packaging, is in fact prescribing a drug and therefore practising medicine?

I don't believe any reasonable person would seriously argue this. Unfortunately, as I was unable to locate any court decisions expressly dealing with this question, this conclusion cannot be ruled out. Notwithstanding, I believe if we move beyond the bare language of the *Foods and Drugs Act* a more reasoned argument can be developed that supports the conclusion that Holistic Nutritionists who make health claims about food and nutritional supplements in the course of their nutritional counselling practices should not be seen to be prescribing drugs and thereby crossing the threshold into the practice of medicine.

First, in those provinces where "drug" is not defined, rather than looking exclusively to the *Food and Drugs Act*, I believe it is better to look to the rules of other provinces where the term "drug" is defined, because definitions should be considered within the context of the rules in which they are used. The *Food and Drugs Act* exists to protect consumers from fraudulent product claims and to ensure the safety of the products we consume. This is a very different mandate than Professional Exclusivity under a medical act which, as we saw in earlier chapters, is intended to ensure that only individuals with requisite training can perform the activities of a physician. So what federal Parliament may want to call a "drug" for the purpose of controlling manufacturing, labelling and advertising, a provincial legislature may not want to regard as a "drug" for the purposes of determining whether someone is practicing medicine. In this regard it is relevant to note that many substances that are classified as drugs under the *Food and Drugs Act*, are unscheduled over-the-counter medications which anyone of any age is free to purchase.

As we saw earlier, in provinces where the Regulated Health Profession legislation does define the word "drug," it consistently means a substance that is illegal or controlled—such as narcotics, and prescriptions and medications that are sold under the supervision of a pharmacist, and not substances that are historically viewed to be food, or over-the-counter supplements that are available without restriction.

Second, even if we look at the definitions contained in the *Food and Drugs Act*, we really must look at how the words "food" and "drug" are interpreted and applied by Health Canada, and not just to the plain language of the Act. The definitions in the *Food and Drugs Act* were drafted very broadly to give Health Canada a fair amount of flexibility when classifying consumable products. So much turns upon Health Canada's exercise of its discretion.

In response to the huge growth in the market for natural health products, Health Canada used its broad mandate to develop a new regulatory regime known as the *Natural Health Products Regulations*. The purpose of these regulations is to create an appropriate regulatory regime for natural substances that are marketed and sold for their curative or preventive properties, and that would otherwise be classified and regulated as drugs. This regulation essentially defines a Natural Health Product to be:

"a substance set out in Schedule 1 [ed. essentially, a plant or plant material, an alga, a bacterium, a fungus or a non-human animal material] or a combination of substances in which all the medicinal ingredients are substances set out in Schedule 1, a homeopathic medicine or a traditional medicine, that is manufactured, sold or represented for use in

(a) the diagnosis, treatment, mitigation or prevention of a disease, disorder or abnormal physical state or its symptoms in humans;

(b) restoring or correcting organic functions in humans; or

(c) modifying organic functions in humans, such as modifying those functions in a manner that maintains or promotes health."

As a result of this regulation, natural health products while technically "drugs" under the *Food and Drugs Act*, are regulated by Health Canada as a different subset of product altogether:

In Canada, natural health products and foods are regulated under the Food and Drugs Act (FDA) and its associated regulations. Products that meet the definition "natural health product" in the Natural Health Products Regulations (NHPR) are subject to the FDA as it applies to a drug and to the NHPR. Products that are foods as defined in the FDA are subject to the FDA as it applies to food and to Parts A, B and D of the Food and Drug regulations (FDR). A product, that is both a natural health product and food is subject to the NHPR but is exempted from the FDR as they apply to food.[35]

Of particular interest to Holistic Nutritionists, Health Canada has also published a guidance document for understanding the differences between the classification of an item as food, verses as a Natural Health Product.[36] I have summarized below the 4 key differentiators taken into consideration:

1.  **Composition** – When food or an ingredient is present in a product solely to provide nourishment, nutrition or hydration, or to satisfy hunger, thirst or a desire for taste, texture or flavour this is an indication that the product is food. A product that is or

---

[35] Health Canada, *Classification of Products at the Food – Natural Health Product Interface: Products in Food Formats* [online], Natural Health Products Directorate, Food Directorate, June 2010 version 2. http://www.hc-sc.gc.ca/dhp-mps/prodnatur/legislation/docs/food-nhp-aliments-psn-guide-eng.php#A4.
[36] Ibid.

that contains an added ingredient that has no known food purpose but that has only a therapeutic use is likely to be classified a Natural Health Product.

2. **Representations** – Claims that speak to a product having therapeutic uses that are not based on the use of the product as food suggest the product is a Natural Health Product.

3. **Format** – Natural health products are typically sold in a format that allows them to be consumed in measured or controlled amounts (doses). If a product is sold in a particular food format (e.g., a beverage) that lends itself to dosing (e.g., sold in single dosage units or it is sold with a measure that indicates it to be consumed in controlled amounts) this is one indication that the product is a Natural Health Product

4. **Public Perception and History** – If a product has a historical pattern of use as food or if the public perception associated with the use of a product in the marketplace is that it is food, these are indications that the product is food rather than a Natural Health Product. Conversely, if the public perception associated with a product and its history and pattern of use indicate it is sold for a therapeutic purpose this supports the conclusion that the product is a Natural Health Product.

For Holistic Nutritionists who reside in provinces that regulate using the Professional Exclusivity framework there are several factors to be taken into account when recommending over the counter medications, Natural Health Products and food and herbs to clients. First, do not make such recommendations in the context of providing a treatment for a disease or disorder unless you live in a province where this may lawfully be done. Second, consult a lawyer and/or review the rules in your province to determine whether "drug" is defined. Third, if the rules do not define what is or is not a drug, consider whether the substance would be a drug in a province that does provide a definition. For example, in provinces that regulate using the Restricted Activity framework, the restriction on prescribing drugs tends to refer to substances that are illegal or controlled—such as narcotics, and prescriptions and medications that are sold under the supervision of a pharmacist. Fourth, consider whether the substance you are recommending is truly food. If it is food and not a drug under the *Food and Drugs Act*, there is a very strong argument that the substance is also not a drug for the purpose of practicing medicine, even if it does contain healing or medicinal properties. Finally, consider whether the substance is a Natural Health Product under Canada's *Food and Drugs Act*. Such products are regulated under as a unique product class under the *Natural Health Products Regulations* notwithstanding the fact they would otherwise be classified as drugs, under this Act. It is also useful to note that in certain provinces, such as Ontario, Natural Health Products are expressly excluded from the definition of "drugs" for the purpose of Restricted Activities.

While I cannot say for certain that a court will never find a Holistic Nutritionist to have prescribed a drug when recommending an over the counter medication, Natural Health Product, or food or herbs with healing properties, I do believe a strong argument can be advanced that these substances are not and should not be viewed to be drugs in the context of determining whether someone is engaged in the practice of medicine.

## Practice of Medicine

The provinces of Manitoba[37], New Brunswick, Nova Scotia, Prince Edward Island, Newfoundland and Labrador, and Saskatchewan currently use a Professional Exclusivity framework and prohibit unauthorized persons from engaging in the practice of medicine.

If the province in which you practice regulates by restricting the practice of medicine, you should review the rules to determine whether any specific activities are restricted. For example, Manitoba and Saskatchewan expressly define the practice of medicine to include diagnosing and treating diseases and disorders and other specific activities. You should also be aware that where such activities are identified, they are not typically exhaustive. By this I mean the rules also leave it open for the courts to decide whether any other procedures and activities should also constitute the practice of medicine.

So, in addition to any specific procedures identified within applicable rules as being an aspect of the practice of medicine, what other activities should be avoided?

If you practice in one of the provinces that regulate using the Professional Exclusivity framework, I believe the safest approach is to avoid engaging in any activities other provinces have deemed to be Restricted Activities, or included within their definition of "practice of medicine." The reader can develop a complete list of these activities and procedures by reviewing the legislation summaries for the provinces set out in Chapter 3. I have also set out below an edited list that includes the activities and procedures I believe Holistic Nutritionists should be particularly aware of because they either involve an aspect of nutritional counselling or are activities an unaware practitioner could engage in while trying to help a client.

1. Advertising, holding out to the public or representing in any manner that you are authorized to practice medicine.

---

[37] It is anticipated by the The College of Physicians and Surgeons of Manitoba that it will transition over to the new Restricted Activity framework sometime in 2015. "The College" Volume 49, Number 3 December 2013.

2.  Offering or undertaking to prevent or to diagnose, correct or treat in any manner or by any means, methods, devices or instrumentalities any disease, illness, pain, wound, fracture, infirmity, defect or abnormal physical or mental condition of any person.

3.  Ordering or receiving reports of screening or diagnostic tests.

4.  Performing a procedure on tissue below the skin, etc.

5.  Inserting or removing an instrument or a device, hand or finger into a body opening.

6.  Administering a substance by injection, inhalation, etc.

7.  Prescribing, compounding or dispensing or administering a drug or vaccine.

8.  In relation to a therapeutic diet that is administered by enteral instillation or parenteral instillation:
    a.  selecting ingredients for the diet; or
    b.  compounding or administering the diet.

9.  Performing a psycho-social intervention with an expectation of modifying a substantial disorder of thought, mood, perception, orientation or memory that grossly impairs judgment, behaviour, the capacity to recognize reality, or the ability to meet the ordinary demands of life.

10. Allergy challenge testing or allergy desensitizing treatment involving injection, scratch tests or inhalation, and allergy challenge testing by any means with respect to a patient who has had a previous anaphylactic reaction.

Over the years, various courts in Canada have looked at the activities that may or may not constitute the practice of medicine. I have summarized below key points identified in some of these decisions along with brief quotations from the judges to help you get a better feel for how the courts look at the practice of medicine.

•   There can be no definitive definition of medicine:

    Nevertheless, we cannot say that the profession, wide as have been its conquests and extended the scope of its practice, has taken all knowledge of the art of healing for its province, and therefore the question submitted (in its alternative form) does not admit of a universal answer in the affirmative. We can only say that the words to practice medicine may include cases in which the remedy prescribed, etc., does not involve the use of drugs or other substances. Every case must stand and be determined upon its own facts and circumstances. We cannot lay down a rule or formulate an answer which will include all.[38]

- The practice of medicine is broader than merely prescribing drugs and medication:

'Practising medicine' is not a definite and finally established term. There is much room for argument both as to what should be called 'medicine' and as to what should be called 'practising'. . . . The term 'practising medicine' need not and does not, in my opinion, necessarily involve only the prescribing or administering of a drug or other medicinal substance, but may well include all such means and methods of treatment or prevention of disease as are from time to time generally taught in the medical colleges and practiced by the regular or registered practitioner. . . .[39]

- The practice of medicine involves monetary gain:

A person in order to render himself liable for practising medicine under the *Medical Act* [R.S.O. 1897, c. 176, s. 49], must have, for gain, prescribed or recommended for trial a particular remedy selected by himself as appropriate to the symptoms described by the patient.[40]

- Suggesting possible remedies and speaking to their properties may not constitute the practice of medicine if the client makes the final decision:

If the patient selects a remedy for himself, making up his own mind as to what he ought to take, there is no offence. A druggist is allowed, it appears, to state fully the qualities and properties of two or more remedies, and even to say which in his opinion is the better remedy or compound, but he must stop short of recommending which remedy the patient had better take for his alleged trouble or complaint.[41]

- The practice of medicine involves more than an isolated activity:

The single act of prescribing medicine to one person on one day will not amount to a practising of medicine . . . Evidence of acts of practising antecedent . . . and possibly . . . subsequent to the date laid in the conviction . . . might be given . . . as establishing . . . a practising of medicine. These acts, however, must be sufficiently approximate in point of

---

[38] Ontario Medical Act, Re (1906) 13 O.L.R. 501
[39] Ibid.
[40] R. v. Coulson as cited in R. v. Valleau, (1900) 3 C.C.C. 435
[41] Ibid.

time to afford evidence of practising, rather than tending to establish the commission of a separate offence.[42]

The words of the Act appear to me to point rather to an habitual, or at all events a continuous course of conduct, than to an isolated act as constituting the offence.[43]

- An isolated act may be sufficient for a practice, if there is also the intention to carry on a business:

It was stated in the judgment of this Division in Rex v. Cruikshanks (1914) 6 W.W.R. 524, at 526, 7 Alta. L.R. 92, at 96, 23 C.C.C. 23, that: "There is no doubt that the law does not contemplate a single act as constituting the practice of a profession or trade," but it was also pointed out by Beck, J., in Rex v. Stimmel, [1923] 3 W.W.R. 1185, at 1201, 19 Alta. L.R. 719, at 738, that "a single or isolated act coupled with an intent to carry on business would suffice." [44]

- Notifying a client that you are not a doctor is not determinative. It is what is done that matters.

Windrum argued that his acts were either not intended or not perceived as practising medicine. In my view that is not relevant. The issue before the court is whether he was practising medicine. In other words, was he diagnosing or treating patients. The learned trial judge concluded that Windrum was practising medicine and in my view there was overwhelming evidence to support that finding.[45]

If the province in which you practice restricts the practice of medicine, the definitions for Diagnosis, Diseases & Disorders, Drugs, and Treatment should also be reviewed, as these are all aspects of practising medicine.

## Treatment

The meaning of what it is to "treat" a disease or disorder is important both in provinces where the practice of medicine is restricted, (as the act of treating a disease or disorder is consistently interpreted to be an aspect of practising medicine) as well as in provinces in which the act of administering a treatment is a Restricted Activity. Here are some of the ways "treatment" has been defined:

---

[42] R. v. Lee (1901) 3 C.C.C. 435
[43] Apothecaries Co. v. Jones (1893) 1 Q.B. 89
[44] R. v. Burton, (1939) 2 D.L.R. 526
[45] R. v. Windrum

The medical or surgical management of a patient.[46]

To manage a disease by medicinal, surgical or other measures; to care for a patient medically or surgically. [47]

The action or management of treating a patient medically or surgically. The management and care of a patient for the purpose of combating disease or disorder.[48]

The Sandhar decision was previously reviewed in connection with the meaning of "diagnoses." However, in this case Mr. Sandhar was also found guilty of prescribing a treatment by virtue of recommending a liver cleanser to address the liver inflammation he diagnosed. As with the diagnosis, it is very unlikely a doctor practising in Alberta at the time would have prescribed the same treatment as Mr. Sandhar; however, this fact did not impact the decision. What mattered to the court was whether the substance was intended to prevent or alleviate a disease or disorder:

> The Respondent is also in contravention of s. 76 in that pursuant to the definition in practising medicine in s. 77 of the Act, he prescribed or administered a treatment for the prevention, alleviation or cure of any human disease or ailment. In particular, the Respondent sold to Miss Lewis for the sum of $10.00 a liver cleanser which was to alleviate or eliminate the problem she had with liver inflammation.[49]

This point was made even more clearly in the R. v. Kish decision involving two phytologists who prescribed hydrogen peroxide as a cure for lung cancer:

> Counsel for the accused argued that the Crown had failed to call any expert evidence to the effect that what the Kishes were doing fell within the purview of medical practice as understood by practising physicians in the Province of Alberta. In fact, it is argued by counsel for the accused that because Dr. Hoy testified for the Crown that the type of treatments being prescribed by the Kishes were not recognized by the medical profession, that this type of activity therefore fell outside of the bounds of ss. 76 and 77 of the Medical Profession Act. . . . With respect I disagree and find that regardless of the philosophical view one takes of the Medical Profession Act, the evidence of Dr. Hoy was clearly to the effect that the treatment of cancer fell squarely within his purview and other duly qualified members of the medical profession.

---

[46] William R. Hensyl, ed., *Stedman's Medical Dictionary,* 25th ed. (Baltimore: Williams & Wilkins, 1990).
[47] Ibid.
[48] Ibid.
[49] R. v. Sandhar

> On the basis of all of the evidence there is no doubt in my mind that what the Kishes did was prescribe a course of treatment clearly directed at and purporting to be able to cure the cancer that Pollock suffered from. By whatever definition of "treatment" is used (and I would refer specifically to those definitions used by Cooke J. in *R. v. Ringrose* (1989), 94 A.R. 350 (Q.B.), at p. 353) the prescribing of hydrogen peroxide to be taken internally for the purpose of killing cancer cells and curing cancer falls squarely within even the narrowest interpretation of "treatment." [50]

Finally, the decision in <u>R. v.Windrum</u> showed prescribing vitamins as a treatment still constitutes prescribing a medical treatment:

> Dr. Loewen, who was qualified as an expert, said that the diagnosis is a conclusion about the patient's condition based on her history, physical examination and tests if necessary. He went on to state that one can diagnose by examining the patient's blood. Furthermore, many of the conditions found by Windrum could be diagnosed by following the above process. In Dr. Loewen's opinion it was common practice to treat patients by prescribing vitamins or iron supplements. [51]

Once again, as with other definitions, we see that the term "treatment" is broadly interpreted and is not restricted to a particular process or modality. When trying to decide whether your actions constitute prescribing or administering a treatment, the key issue to focus upon is whether you are attempting to manage a disease or disorder, not whether the treatment itself is recognized by medicine.

Nor is the question of prescribing treatment linked to the safety of the remedy prescribed. To return to examples I have used elsewhere in this book, scurvy is an illness and dehydration is a disorder. Prescribing vitamin C to remedy scurvy and water to remedy dehydration, while seemingly harmless prescriptions, constitutes prescribing treatment. It does not matter that the substance is not a drug, is safe and widely consumed; what matters is that in making the recommendation you are attempting to manage a disease or disorder.

Finally, when considering the restrictions that relate to recommending a treatment, we must look at a prohibition that exists in *Food and Drugs Act* and that applies within all provinces, even where it is otherwise lawful for Holistic Nutritionists to prescribe treatments.

Section 3 of the *Food and Drugs Act* provides:

---

[50] <u>R. v. Kish</u>
[51] <u>R. v.Windrum</u>

3. (1) No person shall advertise any food, drug, cosmetic or device to the general public as a treatment, preventative or cure for any of the diseases, disorders or abnormal physical states referred to in Schedule A.

(2) No person shall sell any food, drug, cosmetic or device

(a) that is represented by label, or

(b) that the person advertises to the general public

as a treatment, preventative or cure for any of the diseases, disorders or abnormal physical states referred to in Schedule A.

The Act broadly defines "advertisement" to be "any representation by any means whatever for the purpose of promoting directly or indirectly the sale or disposal of any food, drug, cosmetic or device." The current list of Schedule "A" diseases and disorders is reasonably long and includes such common maladies as asthma and obesity. Here is the complete list:[52]

| | |
|---|---|
| Acute alcoholism | Gangrene |
| Acute anxiety state | Glaucoma |
| Acute infectious respiratory syndromes | Haematologic bleeding disorders |
| Acute, inflammatory and debilitating arthritis | Hepatitis |
| Acute psychotic conditions | Hypertension |
| Addiction (except nicotine addiction) | Nausea and vomiting of pregnancy |
| Appendicitis | Obesity |
| Arteriosclerosis | Rheumatic fever |
| Asthma | Septicemia |
| Cancer | Sexually transmitted diseases |
| Congestive heart failure | Strangulated hernia |
| Convulsions | Thrombotic and Embolic disorders |
| Dementia | Thyroid disease |
| Depression | Ulcer of the gastro-intestinal tract |
| Diabetes | |

In the report of the Standing Committee on Health[53] delivered to the House of Commons in 1998, the purpose of this blanket prohibition was identified as being "to ensure individuals will

---

[52] *Food and Drugs Act.*
[53] Canada. Parliament. House of Commons. Standing Committee on Health. *Natural Health Products: A New Vision.* 36th Parliament, 1st Session. (November, 1998).

seek medical attention for serious diseases, to restrict advertising when self-diagnosis and self-treatment is not considered advisable and to limit the possibility of fraudulent claims being made with respect to food and drugs." The committee found these provisions to be unduly restrictive to the detriment of consumers, and recommended that Health Canada investigate whether the prohibition should either be eliminated or amended by more tightly defining and/or removing diseases from Schedule "A."

Notwithstanding the Standing Committee's views, section 3 and Schedule "A" of the *Food and Drugs Act* remains in force today. For Holistic Nutritionists who are otherwise permitted to prescribe treatments in their province, the key difficulty with the Act is the breadth of its definitions, which at first blush appear to restrict the making of any representations or claims (i.e., advertisement) about the curative or preventive value of food (carrots?) and drugs (which would include Natural Health Products) for any Schedule "A" listed disease even if done in the course of a legitimate nutritional consulting practice.

The good news is that the restriction is not quite this tight.

First, the prohibition relates to product labels and to advertising. Since labels are affixed by manufacturers, the concern for Holistic Nutritionists is with advertising, and the definition of advertising clearly states that the representation must be made for the purpose of promoting the sale or disposal of food, drugs, etc. As a result, only Holistic Nutritionists who are involved directly or indirectly in retailing food and supplements can be caught by this prohibition. Holistic Nutritionists who recommend the consumption of certain food or Natural Health Products and who are not involved in their sale or receiving a commission from the retailer are not engaged in "advertising" (and therefore will not breach the *Food and Drugs Act*) even if their comments extend to representations about the preventive or curative properties of products in relation to a Schedule "A" disease or disorder.

Second, out of a concern that the prohibition against advertising contained in Section 3 of the *Food and Drugs Act* was too broad and contrary to the best interests of consumers, an exception was introduced into the regulations to permit the advertising of preventive claims (but not curative or treatment claims) about Drugs[54] and Natural Health Products[55]. As a result, even Holistic Nutritionists who are directly involved in retailing Natural Health Products may make representations about their ability to prevent (but not cure or treat) Schedule "A" diseases and disorders. Food is not specifically mentioned in the regulations because, as previously discussed when defining the word "Drug," a substance that is typically viewed to be "Food" is regulated

---

[54] Sections A.01.067 and A.01.068, Food and Drug Regulations (C.R.C., c. 870)
[55] Section 103.2 and 103.3 Natural Health Products Regulations SOR/2003-196

under the *Food and Drugs Act* as a "Drug" when a representation is made about preventive or curative properties.

Finally, it is important to note that sections 5(1) and 9(1) of the *Food and Drugs Act* also prohibit, among other things, advertising or selling food or drugs in a manner that is "false, misleading or deceptive or is likely to create an erroneous impression regarding its character, value, quantity, composition, merit or safety."

Holistic Nutritionists who are otherwise permitted to prescribe treatments for diseases and disorders within their provinces and who are involved in retailing food, drugs or Natural Health Products to the general public, must be careful not to (1) make any representations about the curative and treatment qualities of the items they are selling in respect of the diseases and disorders listed in Schedule "A" to the *Food and Drugs Act*, or (2) make any false, misleading or deceptive claims about its character, value, quantity, composition, merit or safety.

# Chapter 5
# Pulling It All Together

In this book we have looked at some of the reasons why the provision of health services including nutritional health services is regulated, the different approaches used by the provinces for regulation, specific rules that are in place within each province that impact upon a Holistic Nutrition practice, the meanings of key terms used in these rules, and examples from real cases where people have been charged with unlawful practice of medicine for providing health services that included nutritional advice. This chapter will build upon this foundation to develop some concrete rules Holistic Nutritionists can look to in managing their practices to stay on the right side of the law.

## Choose a Lawful Professional Title

In health services, professional titles matter a great deal. They are seen as the primary means by which a profession identifies itself to the public and by which the public identifies the unique education and expertise of a profession's members. Impersonation of a physician (i.e., the wrongful use of professional titles reserved for the medical profession) is the most common reason cited by many Colleges of Physicians and Surgeons for an unlawful practice prosecution. In health services, every province has created and enforces lists of professional titles that are reserved for use by members of designated Regulated Health Professions. They do, however, approach this issue differently.

Some provinces, such as Ontario, reserve only a very narrow range of specific titles, such as "Physician" and "Dietitian." Others have lengthy lists that include English and French versions, short forms and other common variations of a main title. For example, Nova Scotia reserves the following titles for use by Registered Dietitians: "Dietitian" or "Dietician"; "Dietitian-Nutritionist"; "Nutritionist"; "Professional Dietitian" or "Professional Dietician"; "Professional

Dietitian-Nutritionist"; "Professional Nutritionist"; "Diététiste"; "Diététiste-Nutritionniste"; "Diététiste Professionelle"; "Diététicienne"; "Nutritionniste" or the initials "P.Dt." or "Dt.P."

Finally, some provinces, in addition to the foregoing, also maintain a general prohibition against using any title that wrongly implies membership in a Regulated Health Profession. In Quebec, for example if you are not a member of the "Ordre professionnel des diététistes du Québec" you may not "take or use any name, title, or description implying or calculated to lead people to infer that the person is a registered dietitian."

Holistic Nutritionists must know the rules that restrict the use of professional titles within the province in which they practice.

As a rule of thumb, a Holistic Nutritionist may use a professional title if it accurately describes his or her education, professional qualifications and practice, is not reserved for use by a Regulated Health Profession, and is otherwise lawfully available for them to use[56]. Where a professional title is restricted (such as "Nutritionist" in Nova Scotia) the safest approach is to also avoid using all equivalent versions of the title in other languages, and all short forms, abbreviations and common variations. Finally, a Holistic Nutritionist should avoid using any professional title that could reasonably be seen as implying he or she is a member of a Regulated Health Profession.

As for the most common titles to avoid, Holistic Nutritionists in all provinces should avoid using any title associated with the medical professions (e.g., Doctor, Dr., MD., Surgeon, Physician, etc.), naturopathy (e.g., Naturopath, Naturopathic Doctor, etc.) and the title "Dietitian," which is reserved for use by registered Dietitians in all Canadian provinces. In addition, Holistic Nutritionists practising in Alberta, Nova Scotia and Quebec should avoid using the title "Nutritionist" plus, of course, as mentioned above, all common variations, abbreviations, and non-English equivalents.

## Avoid Using Medical Terms

Many of the rules dealing with professional titles also prohibit any advertisement or claim that is intended to wrongly indicate an ability to diagnose or treat diseases, or membership in a Regulated Health Profession. Holistic Nutritionists should avoid using terms that are associated with the practice of medicine and other Regulated Health Professions in their advertising, marketing literature and client documents. For example, terms such as: registered, medical, medicine, naturopathic, homeopathic, patients, diagnostic, treatment, and their common

---

[56] For example, the professional designations of the Canadian Association of Natural Nutritional Practitioner may only be used by individuals who are member of this organization in good standing.

variations should be avoided. In general, any phrase that could lead a reasonable person to wrongly believe you are a physician, dietitian, naturopath (where this is a Regulated Health Profession) or member of another Regulated Health Profession should be avoided.

## Avoid Diagnosing Diseases and Disorders

Every province with the exception of Alberta either directly or indirectly[57] reserves the act of diagnosing diseases and disorders to specific Regulated Health Professions. This means Holistic Nutritionists in every province other than Alberta must be careful not to render a diagnosis. This can be difficult. There is nothing more natural, and perhaps more intuitive, when dealing with a client than inquiring into health history and complaints and making suggestions for improvement. How can this be done safely? Here are some suggestions:

- Restrict enquiries and activities to evaluating degrees of health. Medicine approaches health from the perspective of identifying and curing diseases. Where there are no diseases or abnormal conditions, health is considered to be present. By contrast, Holistic Nutritionists seek to investigate and enhance health. The act of identifying dietary and nutritional habits that can be changed to improve overall health does not constitute diagnosing diseases and disorders.

- Avoid reaching conclusions based on symptomology. If a disease or disorder is suspected, the client should be told of this suspicion and told to consult a doctor. Never render a verdict or make a conclusion about a client's health. Do not say "You have cancer" or "low blood sugar" or "an iron deficiency." A diagnosis is a conclusion about health and is not something Holistic Nutritionists are typically trained to do.

- When reporting a suspected disease or disorder to a client, put it in writing so there is clear evidence that the client was (1) notified of a suspicion, (2) informed a suspicion is not a diagnosis or conclusion about the state of his or her health, and (3) directed to consult a doctor.

- Do not diagnose symptoms. Do not link symptoms to diseases.

- Emphasize educating clients about good nutrition. Empower clients to make their own conclusions about their health.

---

[57] I consider rendering a diagnosis to be indirectly restricted in any province where the practice of medicine is restricted, as it is clear from case law that the practice of medicine includes diagnosing human diseases and disorders.

- Have clients list all known diseases and disorders on their in-take forms. If a client reveals a disease or disorder, you are not making a diagnosis.

- Do not order blood and other medical diagnostic tests or collect specimens from the human body.

- Never second-guess a diagnosis made by a doctor or other Regulated Health Professional. If an error is suspected, encourage the client to obtain a second opinion from another licensed practitioner.

- Whenever possible, practice in conjunction with a physician or naturopath or a member of another appropriate Regulated Health Profession in your province.

- Be aware of the enforcement practices of regulators and their threshold for enforcement.

Holistic Nutritionists who practice in Alberta are permitted to make a diagnosis. However, as this is not a skill Holistic Nutritionists are typically trained to perform, you should venture down this path very carefully, and only if properly trained. Performing a diagnosis in Alberta may be legal, but you can still cause great harm if wrong and be sued by a client for malpractice if negligent.

## Avoid Treating Diseases and Disorders if Practising Outside Alberta and Ontario

Different provinces take different positions on the treatment of diseases. At the time this is being written, Holistic Nutritionists who practice within British Columbia, Manitoba,[58] New Brunswick, Newfoundland and Labrador, Nova Scotia, Prince Edward Island, Quebec and Saskatchewan are either directly or indirectly[59] prohibited from prescribing treatments for diseases and disorders.

Holistic Nutritionists who practice within Alberta and Ontario may prescribe treatments for diseases and disorders, provided they do so safely, do not perform a Restricted Activity, and comply with the provisions of the *Food and Drugs Act*, including its prohibition against advertising cures and treatments for diseases and disorders listed in Schedule "A" of the Act.

For Holistic Nutritionists who practice within a province where prescribing a treatment is restricted, what can they do? How do you assist clients to improve health, but not be seen to be prescribing treatment? Here are some suggestions:

---

[58] Once the transition to the Restricted Activity framework is completed the making of a diagnosis will be restricted in Manitoba, but not prescribing a treatment, unless doing so involves another procedure which is restricted.

[59] I consider prescribing a treatment to be indirectly restricted in any province where the practice of medicine is restricted, as it is clear from case law that the practice of medicine includes treating human diseases and disorders.

- Do not claim to "treat" or manage a disease or disorder and do not promise to cure or improve a known health condition. Food and nutritional supplements do not cure diseases or conditions; they strengthen the body and enhance the body's ability to maximize its own health.

- Do not prescribe products, or dietary changes to address a known health condition, unless doing so under the supervision of a Regulated Health Professional, where such joint practices are lawful. The threshold for what constitutes prescribing a treatment is very low. Any attempt to "manage" a recognized disease or disorder, through any means, constitutes treatment, regardless of how safe or common the remedies prescribed.

- Do not second-guess a treatment prescribed by a doctor or other Regulated Health Professional. If an error is suspected, encourage the client to obtain a second opinion from another qualified practitioner.

- Always instruct clients to consult a licensed physician or naturopath (where naturopathy is a Regulated Health Profession) about any suspected disease or disorders.

- Keep a record of a client's doctor and the advice the doctor has provided.

- Emphasize educating clients about good nutrition.

- If possible, practice in conjunction with a physician or naturopath or a member of another appropriate Regulated Health Profession.

- Do not prescribe drugs and medications. This is an aspect of practising medicine, or a Restricted Activity, in all Canadian provinces.

- Do not prescribe homeopathic remedies. Regardless of whether they are considered drugs, they are substances that are designed to treat diseases and disorders.

- Recommend only food or Health Canada approved Natural Health Products.[60] Licensed products can be identified by an eight digit product licence number beginning with the letters "NPN" or "DIN-HM"[61]. Exempt products can be identified by a product code beginning with the letters "EN" until they are phased out.

---

[60] It is illegal in Canada to sell a Natural Health Product unless that product holds a Natural Health Product Licence, or Exemption Number. The issuance of new Exemption Numbers was discontinued as February 2013 and products that rely upon Exemption Numbers are in the process of being transitioned to a license, or phased out.
[61] The DIN-HM designation applies to homeopathic remedies.

- Holistic Nutritionists who sell food, drugs or Natural Health Products must comply with the provisions of the *Food and Drugs Act* which permits the making of preventive claims about the products being sold, but not the making of curative or treatment claims, so far as they relate to diseases and disorders listed in Schedule "A" of the Act.

- Be aware of the enforcement practices of regulators and their threshold for enforcement.

## Practice as a Complimentary Therapy

Holistic Nutrition and other unregulated health providers operate in a part of the industry which is increasingly being known as "complimentary therapies." I like this description because it also describes the safest way to operate your practice: complimentary.

Practicing as a complimentary therapy means recognizing the proper role of nutritional counselling. It is not the role of Holistic Nutritionists to diagnose diseases and disorders, nor to be front line care providers in treating the myriad of illnesses that exist. Generally, unless a Holistic Nutritionist has additional training as a physician, or naturopath, or other licensed practitioner, he or she is not properly trained to perform either of these functions, even where it may be legal to do so. The role of a Holistic Nutritionist is to use nutrition to maximize an individual's health and well-being.

If a client has no diagnosable diseases or disorders, but wants to improve his or her health, this means educating them about better nutritional habits, recommending dietary changes and supplements and helping them to reach their nutritional and health goals. These activities can be lawfully carried out in virtually all Canadian provinces. (see "Know the Practice Restrictions That Apply Within Your Province" below).

If, on the other hand, a client has a disease or disorder this means educating them about better nutritional habits and helping them reach their nutritional goals along-side treatments prescribed by the physician, or naturopath, or other licensed practitioner who is the primary care provider.

Does this mean Holistic Nutritionists are generally free to treat persons with diseases and disorders? The answer is both yes and no.[62] Yes you can provide nutritional counselling services to improve overall health and wellness, or reinforce the immune systems of clients who have diseases and disorders, but no you are not free to treat those diseases or disorders unless you practice in Alberta or Ontario.

---

[62]This discussion does not apply to Holistic Nutritionists practicing in New Brunswick and Nova Scotia, who face tighter restrictions than present in other provinces.

What I am suggesting is that treating a person is not always the same as treating a disease or disorder. You can provide nutritional counselling services to help any individual maximize his or her health and well-being, in whatever state of health they may be in, provided you leave the treatment of known diseases and disorders to licensed physicians, or naturopaths, etc.

Restrict your services to complementing, not replacing, such treatments.

If we go back to the case of R. v. Kish discussed in chapters 1 and 4 you will recall the Kishes were found guilty of practicing medicine because, in the words of the court, "On the basis of all of the evidence there is no doubt in my mind that what the Kishes did was prescribe a course of treatment clearly directed at and purporting to be able to cure the cancer that Pollock suffered from." Had the Kishes not recommended that their client discontinue his chemotherapy treatments, and had the Kishes limited their involvement to improving their client's overall health while allowing his physicians to treat his cancer, I believe the case would have been decided differently, if the Kishes would have been charged at all.

This is the essence of a complimentary therapy approach.

If you reside in a province that restricts you from treating diseases and disorders, you can still work to improve the health of your clients who are fighting diseases and disorders. But you should: (1) ensure your client is seeing and receiving treatment from a physician, naturopath, or other licensed practitioner for any known illness, (2) refrain from criticizing, second guessing or otherwise commenting on the treatments, (3) work cooperatively with this professional, or at a minimum ensure they are informed of your role as a nutritional advisor, and (4) focus your efforts and nutritional knowledge on improving your client's over-all health and immune system, apart from the disease.

## Know the Practice Restrictions That Apply Within Your Province

As mentioned may times throughout this book, the provision of health services is regulated provincially. What is lawful in one province may not be lawful in another. Holistic Nutritionists must know the rules that exist within the province in which they practice and avoid relying upon chat groups and discussion forums for guidance.

Holistic Nutritionists who practice in Alberta, B.C., Manitoba, Ontario or Quebec must know and avoid all Restricted Activities within their province. Holistic Nutritionists practising in the other provinces must avoid any activity that is included within the scope of the practice of medicine. This is crucial because "practice of medicine" is broadly defined by the courts, and as we have seen, includes among other activities, diagnosing and treating diseases and disorders.

Of particular relevance for Holistic Nutritionists are rules that regulate the provision of nutrition and dietary management services, because these are closest in nature to what Holistic Nutritionists do. For example, in Quebec common sense may tell you that "providing pregnancy care and conducting deliveries" are Restricted Activities. However, a Holistic Nutritionist practising in Quebec must also be aware that only a member of the Ordre professionnel des diététistes du Québec (or another Regulated Health Plan that is similarly authorized) may: "(a) determine a nutritional plan, including the appropriate feeding route, where an individual prescription indicates that nutrition is a determining factor in the treatment of illness; and (b) monitor the nutritional status of persons whose nutritional treatment plan has been determined." Similarly, Holistic Nutritionists practising in British Columbia should be aware that only registered dietitians may "design, compound or dispense therapeutic diets if nutrition is administered through enteral means."

Holistic Nutritionists practising within the provinces of New Brunswick, Nova Scotia and Manitoba need to exercise particular caution. In New Brunswick the *Dietitians Act* restricts virtually all nutritional counselling to registered dietitians and other similarly authorized Regulated Health Professions. In Nova Scotia the new Medical Act contains an extremely broad definition of practice of medicine that introduces considerable uncertainty as to the scope of what may be lawfully done. This situation will be further aggravated when the new *Dietitians Act* is proclaimed into force. In Manitoba it is arguable that nutritional counselling is presently reserved for registered naturopaths, at least until their regulation is transitioned to this province's new *Health Professions Act*.

In all cases, readers should refer back to the rules in place within the province in which they practice for a complete list of what may and may not be done.

## Know Your Regulator

From my discussions with several of the provincial Colleges of Physicians and Surgeons, it is clear that enforcement is viewed differently in different provinces. The province of Quebec, for example, is known for strictly enforcing its prohibition against unlawfully diagnosing and prescribing treatment and frequently proceeds against naturopaths (naturopathy is not a Regulated Health Profession in Quebec) and others who provide such advice. This province has a strong consumer protection bias in favour of its Regulated Health Professions. By contrast, the College of Physicians and Surgeons of Saskatchewan maintains an official policy in favour of consumer choice, and informed me that it restricts its enforcement activities to situations of fraud (e.g., where a health service provider impersonates a doctor) and physical harm. The consequence of these two different philosophies is that even though diagnosing and prescribing treatment is directly or indirectly restricted in both provinces, several people are prosecuted each year in Quebec and it has been several years since anyone has been prosecuted in Saskatchewan.

It is crucially important for Holistic Nutritionists to be aware of the enforcement practices within their province.

If it does not make sense to you that provinces enforce their laws differently, consider how speeding is enforced on our highways. If the maximum posted limit is 100 km/hr, travelling at 101 km/hr is illegal and should result in a fine. However, because it is not practical for police to enforce such minor speed violations, they don't begin issuing tickets until a greater violation has occurred, perhaps ten, fifteen or even twenty km/hr over the posted limit. The point at which the police begin to enforce the speed limit depends upon their view of public safety and the practicality of enforcement. On a straight stretch of highway where all the cars are exceeding the posted limit, speeding by five or ten km/hr will likely be ignored. If however, you are passing car after car on a busy section of road or near a school, the same five or ten km/hr infraction may lead to a ticket.

Enforcement practices with respect to health services work in a similar manner. In some provinces regulators recognize different people are attracted to different health modalities and embrace the idea that individuals should be entitled to choose their own health care provider, no matter how unconventional. They enforce their laws accordingly and tend to proceed only in egregious cases of fraud or risky, invasive procedures. Other provinces take a more paternalistic approach and believe it is the regulator's job to determine which modalities are valid and the level of training required for practitioners. These provinces tend to favour Regulated Health Professions over all others and they enforce their laws accordingly. Over time, the laws should change to reflect these underlying viewpoints. But this takes time, political will and money. In the meantime, accommodation is often made through adjusting enforcement practices.

You can learn about the enforcement practices within the province in which you practice by contacting the Colleges of Physicians and Surgeons, Naturopathy and Dietitians. In some provinces, one or more of these bodies are directly responsible for enforcement, while in others they only provide support to the Crown. In either case, they can usually help you better understand how the law is interpreted and enforced, or provide a referral to someone who can.

I often find non-lawyers are hesitant to contact regulators, believing they will put themselves on a watch list if they do. If this is a concern, do not provide your name, or if asked, advise the regulator that you are calling on a no-names basis. Regulators usually have a public education mandate and are more than willing to offer help. It is also important to understand that enforcement practices can change at any time, usually without announcement. So check back frequently.

## Keep Current

Laws change. What is lawful today may not be lawful tomorrow. No matter where you live in Canada, a good continuing education program includes being aware of the changes to the laws that govern health services.

As we have seen in this book British Columbia recently completed the transition to a Restricted Activity regulatory framework, and Manitoba is in the midst of this process. Holistic Nutritionists practising in B.C. should watch for the eventual removal of the general restriction against treating diseases and disorders, which is still in effect as a legacy from that provinces former *Medical Practitioners Act*. Those practising in Manitoba should watch for a similar change when the transition to regulation under the *Regulated Health Professions Act* is completed. Finally, Holistic Nutritionists practising in Nova Scotia must watch how the new *Medical Act* is interpreted and enforced and plan for the eventual proclamation of the new *Dietitians Act* and the restrictions it contains. Once in effect, the *Dietitians Act* will make it virtually impossible for a Holistic Nutritionist to lawfully provide any type of services to clients.

The need to being aware of the changes to the laws applies to the information provided in this book. The rules summarized in this book are current and accurate at the time it was written, but may not be at the time it is read.

## Practice Within the Scope of Your Training

This book has focused on some of the major rules imposed by the various governments of Canada that regulate, in a meaningful way, the practices of Holistic Nutritionists. In addition to complying with the law, however, Holistic Nutritionists must also be careful to practice within the boundaries of their skill and training. A failure to do so can result in harm to clients, (Remember the Kishes, who prescribed internal and external treatments of hydrogen peroxide as a cure for lung cancer?) lead to law suits for malpractice (i.e., professional negligence) and even prosecution for fraud under the *Criminal Code* if your actions involve knowingly making false claims or misrepresenting your skill and training or professional accreditation. This principle should also be carried through to your marketing literature and client materials. Remember, many provinces not only restrict what you can do, but also what you can say about what you do. Never misrepresent or over-promise what can be achieved for clients.

## Use Appropriate Forms and Waivers

As we saw under the discussions of "practice of medicine," "diagnosis" and "treatment" in the last chapter, it really doesn't matter whether you intended to engage in a restricted practice or activity; all that really matters are your actions. Using correct forms, however, can establish a client's expectations and provide evidence about the content and nature of advice. This can be particularly important in provinces where making a diagnosis is restricted (i.e., all provinces other than Alberta) and an assessment of a client leads you to suspect the presence of a disease or disorder, or the client is seeking treatment (where this may lawfully be done) for a disease or disorder that has been self-diagnosed, or diagnosed by a physician.

A good in-take form (or forms) should cover the following points[63] (I have also included a sample assumption of risk and release of liability form at the end of this chapter):

- You are trained in the body's nutritional needs and you are not a licensed physician naturopath or dietitian.

- You are relying upon the truth and accuracy of all information provided to you by the client, including medical history and the presence or absences of diseases, disorders, etc.

- You do not diagnose [in all provinces except Alberta] or treat [all provinces except Alberta and Ontario] diseases or disorders.

- If you suspect a client suffers from a disease or disorder, the client will be notified. However, this should not be seen as a diagnosis or relied upon in any way, and a physician or other appropriate licensed health professional should be consulted.

- The purpose of nutritional counselling is to improve the body's immune system and overall vitality. Dietary changes and other recommendations should not be seen as, or relied upon for, treating diseases or disorder [all provinces except Alberta and Ontario].

- If a client notifies you of a disease, disorder for which they are seeking nutritional treatment, you are relying without independent verification, upon this diagnosis. If they have not done so, they should have it verified by a physician or other appropriate licensed health professional. [Alberta and Ontario only.]

---

[63] It is also important to remember that your collection, storage, use and release of client information must comply with privacy and collection of personal information laws in effect in your province, such as Ontario's *Personal Health Information Protection Act*, and the federal government's *Personal Information Protection and Electronic Documents Act*.

## Join a Good Professional Association

As mentioned at the beginning of the book, Holistic Nutritionists, unlike registered dietitians, physicians, and in some provinces naturopaths, are not members of a Regulated Health Profession. This means there is no governing body overseeing the profession to whom Holistic Nutritionists are accountable and to whom the public can appeal when they have questions or complaints.

The benefit of this is that Holistic Nutritionists are free to structure their practices and provide advice in accordance with their training and beliefs, provided they comply with laws of general application. The problem with this situation, however, is that there are no guidelines establishing what it means to be a Holistic Nutritionist and anyone, regardless of their education or training can claim to practice in this area so long as they do not fraudulently misrepresent their credentials, and, of course, otherwise comply with the law. This makes it difficult for properly trained ethical Holistic Nutritionists to stand out, and for the public to identify them.

In response to this situation, several associations have formed over the years to assist Holistic Nutritionists with their practices and to provide the public with a means of skill validation and accountability. The decision of which association is best for you is a personal one. In the interest of full disclosure, I want to point out right now that I am a director of one of these associations—the Canadian Association of Natural Nutritional Practitioners (CANNP). I believe it does the best job representing the interests of its Holistic Nutritionists, and naturally favour it over the others. Regardless of this, however, if you are deciding among associations, I have the following advice and recommendations:

- Nutritionist associations are not governing bodies and do not confer upon their members the right to practice as a Holistic Nutritionist. You do not need their consent to practice.

- Nutritionist associations exist to serve their members. The only reason to join one is to take advantage of the benefits offered to members.

- Confirm the association is a non-profit corporation. A non-profit corporation is a corporation that has members, not shareholders, and is required by law to use the money it collects from membership fees, etc. to fulfill its mandate. It is not permitted to generate a profit. If an association does not permit its members to elect the association's board of directors, ask questions. Odds are the association is not a "non-profit."

- Make sure the association has comprehensive professional guidelines and rules of practice. In a legal action for malpractice, compliance with professional standards and practices is an available defense. An association's professional guidelines and rules of practice can help ensure their members practice in accordance with professional standards, and serve as evidence that they did.

- There is no legal requirement compelling Holistic Nutritionists to maintain practice liability insurance. Having such insurance is, however, typically required as a condition of membership in a Nutritionist association for two reasons: (1) it protects the member by making money available in the event of a legal action for malpractice, and (2) it protects the member's client by ensuring funds are available for damages in the event they are successful in a legal action for malpractice.

- Make sure the association responds to questions and assists with mentoring. These are the services that help Holistic Nutritionists avoid making professional practice and business mistakes.

## Relax and Enjoy What You Do

Holistic Nutritionists provide invaluable services to the public. Their goal is to make people healthy. What can be better than this? Yes, there are many rules that restrict what can be done. But with the exception of New Brunswick[64] where a conventional Holistic Nutritionist's practice contravenes the exclusive practice area of dietitians, Nova Scotia where the new *Medical Act* creates a similar situation vis a vis physicians and the practice of medicine, and in the short term Manitoba where the *Naturopathic Act* may be a problem until naturopaths become regulated under *The Regulated Health Professions Act*, the rules generally permit nutritional counselling services that educate and promote health and wellness and in many cases (i.e., Alberta, Ontario and soon Manitoba) that treat diseases and disorders.

The truth of the matter is that thousands of Holistic Nutritionists provide their services to the public every day, and based upon the legal research I completed, and the anecdotal evidence I collected from the Colleges of Physicians and Surgeon, Colleges of Dietitians and police forces I contacted while researching this book, actions against nutritional advisors are for the most part rare and primarily relate to egregious situations of practising medicine (e.g., the Kishes) unlawful prescription of treatments, and incidences of fraud, where individuals wrongfully represent themselves to the public as physicians, or the possessors of miracle cures. In short, the quacks, sellers of snake oil and other fraudsters we briefly looked at in the first chapter.

---

[64] Nova Scotia will also be in this group, once its new *Dietitians Act* is proclaimed.

# Appendix 1
# Assumption of Risk and Release of Liability
# For Nutrition Counselling Services

The Assumption of Risk and Release of Liability contains two parts.

The first part deals with the client's assumption of risk. This part of the form is designed to minimize liability by ensuring a client receives notice of certain key facts about the practice of Holistic Nutrition and its limitations. In provinces where use of the title "Nutritionist" is restricted, substitute an acceptable title such as "Advisor" or "Counsellor." References to naturopaths should be included only in provinces where naturopaths are a Regulated Health Profession. In provinces where Holistic Nutritionists are permitted to treat clients, references to treatments can be omitted and the alternative version of paragraph 5 can be used.

The second part of this form is a release of liability. The purpose of a release is to minimize liability by having the client release the practitioner from any liability for any negative consequences that may result from the counselling service.

In relying upon this form the following factors must be taken into account:

- This form is provided to illustrate the types of issues an Assumption of Risk and Release of Liability form may deal with.

- The laws of the provinces of Canada differ. All or part of this form may not be enforceable within a particular province.

- Prior to relying upon this form, it should be reviewed by a lawyer licensed to practice in the province within which it is to be used.

- Clients must be of legal age and sound mind when signing a form of this type. Clients should be encouraged to carefully read, ask questions, and if requested, consult a lawyer about any documents they are asked to sign. Never intimidate or coerce a client into signing a form of this type.

# Assumption of Risk and Release of Liability
# For Nutrition Counselling Services

TO:             [insert name of Holistic Nutritionist] (the "Nutritionist[65]")

DATE:        [insert date]

RE:              Nutrition Counselling Services

The undersigned, _____, hereby acknowledges and agrees as follows:

1.  The purpose of nutrition counselling is to improve the overall health, vitality and well-being of the body through nutritional education and the use of natural food and non-medicinal nutritional supplements. The [Nutritionist] does not diagnose [or treat][66] diseases, disorders or conditions.

2.  The [Nutritionist] is not a licensed dietitian, [naturopath][67] or physician.

3.  As part of the Nutrition Counselling Services, I may be asked to provide information concerning my physical habits, medical history, moods, energy levels, likes and dislikes, lifestyle and diet. This information is collected to enable the [Nutritionist] to (i) assess my knowledge of nutrition, (ii) educate me about the benefits of sound nutritional practices, and (iii) recommend dietary changes to improve my general health, vitality and overall well-being. The [Nutritionist] will hold this information in confidence and will not release or disclose this information to any other person, without my prior consent, except as required by applicable law.

4.  If the [Nutritionist] suspects the existence of a disease, disorder or condition, I will be informed of this suspicion. However, I acknowledge this is not a diagnosis or conclusion about the state of my health and that I am directed to promptly consult a licensed physician [or naturopath] about any suspected problems.

5.  Dietary changes and nutritional supplements suggested by the [Nutritionist] are intended to improve the general health, vitality and well-being of my body and are not recommended for the purposes of treating diseases, disorders or conditions. I am not to alter or discontinue treatments prescribed by a licensed physician, [naturopath], or other

---

[65] In provinces where use of the title "Nutritionist" is restricted, substitute an acceptable title such as "Advisor" or "Counsellor."
[66] Reference to treatment can be omitted in the provinces in which a Holistic Nutritionist is permitted to provide treatments.
[67] Include references to naturopaths only in provinces where naturopaths are a Regulated Health Profession.

licensed health professional without consulting the individual who prescribed the treatment.

– Alternate paragraph 5 –

[IN PROVINCES IN WHICH A HOLISTIC NUTRITIONIST IS PERMITTED TO PROVIDE TREATMENT, THE FOLLOWING CAN BE SUBSTITUTED FOR PARAGRAPH 5 ABOVE] Should I request the [Nutritionist] to recommend dietary changes and/or nutritional supplements to enhance my body's natural ability to resist and/or overcome a known disease, disorder or condition, it is my responsibility to disclose the nature of the disease, disorder or condition and all other relevant details to the [Nutritionist]. If I have not previously consulted a licensed physician [or naturopath] about the disease, disorder or condition, I acknowledge that I am directed to promptly do so. I am not to alter or discontinue treatments prescribed by a licensed physician, [naturopath], or other licensed health professional without consulting the individual who prescribed the treatment.

6.  In providing Nutrition Counselling Services to me, the [Nutritionist] is relying upon the truth, accuracy and completeness of all information I have provided to him/her. Any recommendations I follow for changes in diet, including the use of nutritional supplements, are entirely my responsibility.

In consideration of my participation in the Nutrition Counselling Services, I hereby accept all risk to my health, including injury or death that may result from such participation and I hereby release the [Nutritionist], on my behalf and on behalf of my personal representatives, estate, heirs, next of kin and assigns from any and all costs, claims, causes of action and damages arising from any and all illness or injury to my person, including my death, that may result from or occur as a result of my participation in the Nutrition Counselling Services, whether caused by negligence or otherwise.

I HAVE CAREFULLY READ THIS AGREEMENT AND UNDERSTAND IT TO BE A FULL AND FULL AND FINAL RELEASE OF ALL COSTS, CLAIMS, CAUSES OF ACTION AND DAMAGES OF ANY KIND ARISING FROM OR IN CONNECTION WITH THE NUTRITION COUNSELLING SERVICES.

_____        _____

Client Signature                                          Date

Manufactured by Amazon.ca
Bolton, ON